Nurses' Aid Series

PHARMACOLOGY FO

C000318679

NURSES' AIDS SERIES

Anatomy and Physiology for Nurses
Ear, Nose and Throat Nursing
Geriatric Nursing
Mathematics in Nursing
Medical Nursing
Microbiology for Nurses
Multiple Choice Questions, Book 1
Multiple Choice Questions, Book 2
Multiple Choice Questions, Book 3
Obstetric and Gynaecological Nursing
Paediatric Nursing
Personal and Community Health
Pharmacology for Nurses
Practical Nursing
Practical Procedures for Nurses
Psychiatric Nursing
Psychology for Nurses
Sociology for Nurses
Surgical Nursing
Theatre Technique

Special Interest Texts
Accident and Emergency Nursing
Anaesthesia and Recovery
Room Techniques
Cardiac Nursing
Gastroenterological Nursing
Neuromedical and Neurosurgical
Nursing
Nutrition and Dietetics in Health
and Disease
Ophthalmic Nursing
Orthopaedics for Nurses

NURSES' AIDS SERIES

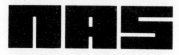

Pharmacology for Nurses

Fifth Edition

James Connechen,
RGN, RMN, RCNT, RNT

Senior Tutor
North West Surrey District School of Nursing

Eamon Shanley,
RMN, RNMH, CPN(Cert), RNT, BA(Hons), MSc

Nursing Research Unit
Dept. of Nursing Studies
University of Edinburgh

Howard Robson,
MA, MB, BChir, MRCP
Consultant Physician
Cumberland Infirmary
Carlisle

BAILLIÈRE TINDALL
LONDON

Published by BAILLIÈRE TINDALL,
a division of Cassell Ltd,
Greycoat House,
10 Greycoat Place
London SW1P 1SB

First published 1964
Third edition 1971
  Reprinted 1972
Fourth edition 1975
  Reprinted 1977
  Reprinted 1978
  Reprinted 1980
  Reprinted 1981
Fifth edition 1983

ISBN 0 7020 0868 0

Spanish edition (CECSA, Mexico) 1973

Designed by Peter Powell MSTD
Typeset by Bookens, Saffron Walden, Essex
Printed in Great Britain by Spottiswoode Ballantyne Ltd
Colchester and London

British Library Cataloguing in Publication Data
Connechen, James
Pharmacology for nurses.—5th ed.—(Nurses'
aids series)
1. Pharmacology   2. Nursing—Study and teaching
I. Title   Shanley, Eamon
III. Robson, Howard
615'.1'024613   RM300
ISBN 0-7020-0868-0

Contents

Preface

We have attempted to maintain Rosemary Bailey's aim of providing an easy to read pharmacology book for nurses, yet with sufficiently detailed information to allow a good understanding of the drugs they use. We have rearranged many of the chapters, lengthened some and reduced others without significantly altering the overall size of the book.

We would like to acknowledge the assistance of Miss Grant, Education Officer, Central Midwives Board for Scotland, in the chapter 'Drugs Used in Midwifery', Dr John Loudon in the chapter, 'Drugs Used in Mental Illness' and Miss Railton, Pharmacist, Cumberland Infirmary, Carlisle. We would also like to thank our respective wives, Jane, Terri and Phyll for their encouragement, and a special thanks to Mrs R. Irwin for her typing skills and good humour. Finally, we would like to mention Rosemary Long of Baillière Tindall for her tolerance and great patience.

July, 1982
James Connechen
Eamon Shanley
Howard Robson

1 Introduction

The use of medicines used to be purely empirical, and their mode of action was unknown. Medicines were often plant extracts, containing many chemical compounds, most of which were inactive. Many preparations had no therapeutic action at all but patients gained a psychological benefit (placebo effect). However, other preparations also contained active ingredients. The ancient Chinese gave 'dragons' teeth' (probably dinosaur teeth) in the treatment of convulsions; today calcium, the main constituent of bone, is given in the treatment of tetany. The remedy for goitre was burnt sponges; a sponge is a marine animal which we now know to contain iodine. A nineteenth-century 'remedy for itch' was 'a mixture of ships' tar and oil'; today we still use purified coal tar as an antipruritic.

The scientific study of therapeutics began in 1785, when William Withering described the use of the Foxglove (containing digitalis). He defined the pathological conditions most likely to respond to treatment, the side effects that might occur, and how the drug should be taken to produce the maximal benefit to the patient with minimal side effects.

Nowadays, drugs are extremely potent, highly purified chemical compounds. Unfortunately, this increases their potential to produce adverse reactions, especially in overdosage.

Of the many new drugs produced by industrial chemists, very few are eventually suitable for patient use. First, a new drug must show a potential therapeutic effect in experimental animals. Further animal studies then assess its toxicity. Next the drug is given to healthy human volunteers to confirm the presence of a useful pharmacological effect in man, and to study what happens to the drug in the human body. If the drug still shows promise, it is given to small, then larger, numbers of volunteers with an illness which might be improved or cured by the drug. The evidence is then put before a Government body (in the UK, the Committee on Safety of Medicines), and if they are satisfied, the drug may be prescribed. Even so, serious adverse reactions necessitating withdrawal of a drug may become apparent only after many years of use.

Before any drug is prescribed for a patient, the probable benefit must outweigh the possible risk. The use of powerful, modern drugs for trivial, self-limiting conditions (such as a 'cold') unnecessarily exposes patients to potential adverse reactions and diverts Health Care finance from more useful areas.

The cost of medicines is variable, but can be considerable. In some instances, a particular brand may cost up to twenty times more for a course of treatment, than a similar, equally effective alternative.

There are pressures on doctors to prescribe unwisely, sometimes from the pharmaceutical industry (who manufacture and sell the drugs) and sometimes from patients themselves, and the nurse must appreciate this. The nurse who understands the action of a drug, its beneficial effects, and its possible adverse reactions, will ensure patients obtain the optimal benefit from modern medicines.

New preparations are constantly appearing and it is impossible for the nurse to be conversant with all of them. The nurse should have a knowledge of the pharmacology of commonly used drugs, their dosage and side effects. Further information about lesser used drugs can be obtained from the British National Formulary and larger clinical pharmacology textbooks. In case of difficulty, enquiry should be made of the doctor or pharmacist.

2 Drugs and the Law

Nurses are involved in drug administration which is controlled by law. Therefore, nurses must understand those aspects of the law which are relevant to their practice.

There are two types of regulation governing the administration of drugs: statutory regulations relating to Acts of Parliament, and local hospital regulations.

LAWS RELATING TO THE CONTROL OF DRUGS

In Great Britain, the storage, administration and sale of drugs are controlled by Acts of Parliament. The aim is to prevent error, improper usage and addiction. These Acts chiefly affect doctors, pharmacists and nurses.

The Medicines Act 1968

This regulates the manufacture, importation, distribution and sale of medicines and veterinary products. It deals with:

1. Product and manufacturing licences (after consultation with the Committee on the Safety of Medicines where appropriate).
2. The registration of retail pharmacies (by the Pharmaceutical Society).
3. Categorization of medicines into three groups, depending on conditions of sale:
   (*a*)Prescription-only medicines, marked POM.
   (*b*)Non-prescription medicines, but limited to pharmacies (Pharmacy Medicines), marked P.
   (*c*)Other outlets permissible (General Sale List), marked GSL.

4. Labelling of medicines.
5. Containers in which they are supplied.
6. Manner in which their role is promoted.

Prescriptions must be written in indelible ink and contain:
  (i) Address and signature of medical practitioner and date.
  (ii) Name, address and age (if less than 12 years) of patient.
  (iii) Name of drug, dosage and frequency of administration (and quantity to be supplied, if not obvious).
Regulations limit the use of repeat prescriptions.

Misuse of Drugs Act 1971

This Act replaced previous Dangerous Drugs Acts, and is concerned with the control of narcotics and other drugs of dependence.

It set up an Advisory Council to review any drug liable to misuse, and to advise the Secretary of State on measures to be taken regarding its manufacture, supply and possession (The Misuse of Drugs Regulations). It also advises on rehabilitation of dependent persons, education of the public, and research.

The Controlled Drugs covered by the Act include: opiates (e.g. morphine, heroin, dipipanone), pethidine, cocaine, phencyclidine, LSD, amphetamines, cannabis, methylphenidate, phenmetrazine and methaqualone, and the injectable preparations of codeine phosphate and dihydrocodeine.

Preparations containing very small amounts of these drugs (e.g. certain cough suppressants) are exempt.

Notification of drug addicts

Doctors must notify patients suspected of addiction to controlled drugs to the Chief Medical Officer.

Prescribing for addicts
Only doctors holding a special licence may prescribe maintenance heroin and cocaine. However, any doctor may
prescribe these drugs for other medical reasons (e.g. pain).

Prescribing controlled drugs
Unless the prescription is completed according to specific
requirements in the Regulations, the pharmacist is not
allowed to dispense controlled drugs. However, in hospital,
the usual patient's prescription sheet is adequate.

Drug abuse can also be reduced by:

1. Avoiding unnecessary prescriptions of potentially addictive
   drugs, e.g. hypnotics.
2. An awareness that addicts will often use devious means
   to obtain drugs, or steal or forge prescriptions.

Containers for controlled drugs
The container must state the formulation (e.g. tablet), strength
of each dose, and the total number of doses. For mixtures and
ointments, the total amount, and proportion of each controlled
drug, must be stated.

Prescribing controlled drugs in hospital
1. Prescriptions must be signed by a registered medical
   practitioner.
2. Stock must be ordered in special Controlled Drug Books,
   and signed by the ward sister (or deputy).
3. Controlled drugs must be delivered in a sealed container
   and a receipt signed by the ward sister.
4. They must be stored in a locked container, within a
   locked cupboard, which must be used for no other
   purpose.
5. Details of each dose given must be recorded in ink in the
   Controlled Drug Book, and signed by the person giving

the dose, and countersigned by the registered or enrolled nurse who checked it.

6. Any drug prepared but not used must be destroyed, recorded and signed for.
7. Controlled Drug Books must be kept for two years following the last entry date.
8. Outdated stock must be returned to the pharmacy.

A State Certified Midwife in domiciliary practice may obtain and administer pethidine, and certain non-controlled drugs, with the approval of the local supervizing authority (see Chapter 19).

LOCAL REGULATIONS FOR ALL DRUGS

These are based on the Aitken Report (1958) and the Gillie Report (1970), and may vary according to local circumstances, but the following guidelines are recommended:

1. Drugs should be checked, prior to administration, by a second nurse.
2. Ward stocks should be as small as practicable, and checked regularly.
3. Drug cupboard keys should be carried by the ward sister (or deputy).
4. Ward drug trolleys should be lockable and, when not in use, locked in a cupboard or by a chain to the wall or floor.
5. Ampoules and boxes containing different drugs should be neatly separated.
6. Drugs requiring refrigeration should be kept in a locked refrigerator.
7. Emergency drugs should be kept on the emergency trolley, preferably in a lockable container fixed to the trolley.
8. Drugs should not be transferred from one bottle to another.

9. Out of date drugs, and those brought in by patients, should be immediately returned to the pharmacy.

10. Preparations intended for external use should be stored in a separate locked cupboard.

11. Additional guidelines are issued to nurses in domiciliary practice regarding the storage, transport and administration of drugs.

12. For nursing responsibilities regarding intravenous injections and additives, see Chapter 25.

3 Basic Clinical Pharmacology and Drug Administration

HOW DRUGS ACT AT A CELLULAR LEVEL

Most drugs chemically resemble an endogenous compound and bind to a specific molecule which may be an enzyme, or part of the cell membrane ('receptor').

Drugs can be either

(*a*) agonists, which activate the receptor, or
(*b*) antagonists, which prevent agonists combining with the receptor.

NOMENCLATURE OF DRUGS

Chemical name
This indicates the molecular structure. Many of these names are complex and unwieldy.

Approved name
An abbreviated form of the chemical name.

Proprietary (brand) name
That given by the company which markets the drug. Since several companies market the same drug, with different proprietary names, unnecessary confusion may arise. When-

ever possible, drugs should be prescribed by their approved names.

Example
Chemical name: acetyl-p-amino-phenol
Approved name: paracetamol
Proprietary names: Calpol, Panadol, Panasorb, Salzone

WEIGHTS AND MEASURES

Weight (mass)
1000 micrograms   =   1 milligram (mg)
1000 milligrams (mg) =   1 gram (g)

Volume
1000 millilitres (ml.)   =   1 litre
1 teaspoon   =   5 ml.

FACTORS INFLUENCING RESPONSE TO DRUG THERAPY

1. Compliance (i.e. does the patient actually take the drugs as prescribed?)
2. Absorption
3. Elimination (inactivation or excretion of the drug by the body)
4. Age
5. Drug interactions
6. Tolerance.

Compliance
Patients are more likely to take medicines as prescribed (especially when out of hospital) if:

(*a*) The benefits are clearly explained.

(*b*) Dosage instructions are clear (preferably written legibly).
(*c*) Treatment is simple (e.g. one tablet once a day).
(*d*) There are no side effects.
(*e*) Relatives and friends are enlisted to help, if memory is poor or if there is a psychiatric disorder.

Absorption
Depends on route of administration:

Oral (as liquid, powder, tablet or capsule). Most convenient, but the rate and extent of absorption may be variable.
Sub-lingual. Tablets allowed to dissolve under the tongue. Rapid action. Some preparations (e.g. trinitrine) are inactivated if swallowed.
Rectal. As suppositories or enemeta. Inconvenient.
Injection
   (*a*) *Intravenous* (i.e. into a vein). Very rapid onset of action, but side effects, such as anaphylaxis, may occur rapidly. Inconvenient.
   (*b*) *Intramuscular.* Usually given into the thigh. Painful, but useful if oral therapy is impracticable.
   (*c*) *Subcutaneous.* Slow absorption.
   (*d*) *Intrathecal.* Given by a doctor into the meningeal space. Now rarely used.
   (*e*) *Epidural.* The injection of drugs just outside the lumbar meninges. Used for local anaesthesia and analgesia.
Inhalation. Usually as aerosol sprays—requires patient dexterity.
Local (topical). Produces high local tissue concentrations of the drug, when only a local effect is required, which minimizes toxicity to the rest of the body. **Examples**: Cutaneous (creams, ointments, lotions), ocular (eye-drops), lungs (aerosols), rectal (suppositories and enemata), and vaginal (pessaries).

Elimination

(*a*) *Metabolism*. Many drugs are inactivated by the liver (e.g. lignocaine). Such drugs may accumulate in liver disease.

(*b*) *Renal excretion*. Other drugs are mainly excreted into the urine (e.g. digoxin, gentamicin). These drugs will accumulate in renal failure. Some drugs are inactivated both by renal excretion and metabolism (e.g. oxprenolol).

Plasma half-life is the time taken for plasma drug concentrations to reduce by half.

Age

Drug elimination is often reduced in the elderly, who are also more sensitive to drug effects.

Drug interactions

Many drugs interfere with absorption, elimination and action of other drugs (e.g. phenobarbitone increases the metabolism of warfarin, thus decreasing its action).

Tolerance

Prolonged administration of some drugs (such as opiates) requires increasing dosage to maintain an effect.

VARIATION OF DOSAGE

Dosage in children should be related to the size of the child.

The elderly usually only tolerate smaller doses.

Owing to incomplete absorption, or metabolism, larger doses are often required when given by mouth, rather than parenterally.

Maximal effects only occur after several doses, unless a higher initial dose is given (loading dose).

Dosage may be adjusted if the drug effect can be measured

(e.g. heart rate for digoxin in atrial fibrillation; prothrombin time for warfarin).

Measurements of plasma drug concentrations are occasionally helpful (e.g. anticonvulsants).

ADVERSE DRUG REACTIONS

These may be due to:

(*a*) Unwanted pharmacological effects (e.g. vomiting with digoxin).
(*b*) Idiosyncrasy, reactions only occurring in certain individuals (e.g. aspirin-induced asthma).
(*c*) Hypersensitivity, due to immunological reactions, the most important being anaphylaxis (asthma and hypotension) which may be fatal within minutes, and blood dyscrasias (e.g. aplastic anaemia).

Liver damage and skin rashes also occur by these mechanisms.

PATIENT EDUCATION

1. Enquire regarding previous adverse drug reactions.
2. Explain reason for drug therapy.
3. Explain dosage regimen.
4. Instruct how to administer (e.g. insulin injections, inhalers).
5. Instruct to report any side-effects.
6. Advise on danger of sudden withdrawal (e.g. corticosteroids).
7. Advise on drug interactions (e.g. warfarin and aspirin).
8. Advise that drugs should be kept away from children.
9. Advise patients to destroy old medicines.
10. Advise patients not to distribute medicines to friends.

ROLE OF THE NURSE IN DRUG TREATMENT

1. Patient education.
2. Ensure compliance.
3. Note any side-effects.
4. Report any change in patient's clinical state.
5. Administer medication:
   (*a*) Only prescribed drugs.
   (*b*) Check therapeutic response if appropriate (e.g. pro-thrombin time for warfarin).
   (*c*) Check drug, dosage, correct time, route of admini-stration and patient's identity in the presence of another nurse. Confirm with doctor if in any doubt.
   (*d*) Record administration on prescription card.
6. Question any prescription which is illegible, appears inappropriate, or may be no longer required.
7. Do not use expired drugs, a solution which has discoloured, a leaking sterile ampoule or infusion bag, or an in-adequately labelled drug.

CONCLUSIONS

The administration of drugs is a specialized nursing skill. The effectiveness of the prescribed drugs is influenced by the nurse's approach to the individual patient. Many patients are highly resistant to 'taking tablets', as drug dependence may be seen as a sign of weakness. The nurse's explanation, sympathetically given in privacy, may allay anxiety. It is important to *listen* to what the patient has to say. He may have a good reason for not complying with recommended treatment.

It is a thoughtful point of technique and good communication if the nurse approaches the patient, sitting down if necessary, to discuss personal problems such as levels of pain, consti-pation, and side-effects from drugs. If pain is discussed at a speaking distance of eight feet, the patient is unlikely to be accurate if he is embarrassed. The drug trolley can be guarded by the witness while the donor listens to the patient.

Nurses will learn the art of drug administration by example and teaching, and find the best and safest ways of, for example, giving an inhalation that is not too hot, serving a warm, soothing linctus, and waiting patiently for tablets to be swallowed. It is imperative to ensure that drugs are taken. If a patient attempts to hide them, the nurse is in a good position to determine why they are not acceptable. The patient who conceals drugs in hospital is unlikely to take them at home.

The process of nursing demands that the nurse's approach to each patient be individual. Mary Jones aged 4 may find ampicillin far less acceptable than does Mrs Brown, who understands why it is needed. As in so many other areas, the nurse must consider patients' unique personal needs in their perception of their illness, and attempt to meet them.

4 Drugs Affecting the Gastro-Intestinal Tract

ANTACIDS AND ULCER-HEALING DRUGS

Antacids produce symptomatic relief of pain associated with peptic ulceration, gastric reflux and oesophagitis. They act by raising the pH value of gastric contents by neutralizing the hydrochloric acid. Since the antacid will be removed during normal gastric emptying, the antacid should have a rapid action and will be required to be taken at frequent intervals. Antacids are obtained in either tablet form to be chewed before swallowing, or in aqueous solution.

Sodium bicarbonate
Dose 1–5 g orally.

Being soluble in water, sodium bicarbonate acts rapidly and so quickly neutralizes hydrochloric acid. Its action, however, is short-lived and any excess of the drug quickly leaves the stomach to be absorbed from the intestine. Prolonged use can therefore cause metabolic alkalosis. It produces carbon dioxide, which will cause gastric distention and eructation of gas. It is not now recommended as an antacid.

Magnesium salts
These are white insoluble powders and therefore not readily

absorbed. Their action is slower and more prolonged than that of sodium bicarbonate. They retain fluid in the bowel, and in large doses cause diarrhoea. This is often counteracted by adding calcium carbonate, which is slightly constipating.

Magnesium hydroxide mixture (*Cream of magnesia*)
Dose 5–10 ml.
   Obtained as a suspension in water. Also used as a mild aperient.

Magnesium carbonate
Dose 250–500 mg.
   May produce carbon dioxide during neutralization.

Magnesium trisilicate mixture
Dose 5–10 ml. orally.
   Slower in effect than other magnesium salts and a larger dose may be required. It is also thought to form a protective adherent gelatinous coat at the base of the ulcer.

Calcium carbonate
A very effective neutralizing agent. Very little is absorbed, but there is a tendency to precipitate in the intestine causing constipation.

Aluminium hydroxide mixture (*Aludrox*)
Dose 5–10 ml.
   A very effective antacid which is also thought to inhibit the action of pepsin. It is given as a tablet to be sucked, or in a colloidal solution. Aluminium hydroxide is not absorbed from the intestine, so it does not cause alkalosis. However, it is slightly astringent and may cause constipation. Alternate aluminium hydroxide and magnesium trisilicate is popular, effective, and causes no bowel upset.

Colloidal bismuth

Tripotassium dicitrato bismuthate (*De-Nol*) and bismuth subnitrate (*Roter*) are effective antacids and ulcer-healing drugs.

Cimetidine (*Tagamet*)

Dosage 400 mg twice daily. A maintenance dose of 400 mg at night will be required for most patients.

Antacids, although neutralizing hydrochloric acid in the stomach, have little influence on the healing of ulcers. Cimetidine is a specific antihistamine acting only on histamine-(H_2) receptor sites in the gastric mucosa. Since histamine stimulates the secretion of hydrochloric acid, cimetidine, by blocking its action, reduces the amount of acid released into the stomach. Unfortunately, discontinuation of the drug often produces a recurrence of the ulcer.

Adverse effects. Drowsiness and a skin rash may occur, while impotence and gynacomastia have been reported.

Ranitidine (*Zantac*)

Dose 150 mg twice daily. Maintenance dose 150 mg at night.

Is an H_2-receptor antagonist like cimetidine.

Carbenoxolone (*Biogastrone*)

Dose 100 mg three times a day for 4–8 weeks.

Carbenoxolone is derived from liquorice and increases the rate of healing of gastric ulcers. Its mode of action is unknown.

Adverse effects. It can cause sodium and water retention and potassium loss, which may lead to oedema, hypertension and hypokalaemia. It is contraindicated in cardiac failure and hypertension.

Duogastrone is a slow-release form of carbenoxolone used in the treatment of duodenal ulcers.

Pyrogastrone contains carbenoxolone, antacids and alginic acid. It is a most effective treatment for oesophagitis: dose, one tablet chewed after meals and two at bedtime.

Dimethicone (*Asilone*)
Dose 5–10 ml. before meals and at night. Also available as tablets.

A defoaming agent claimed to relieve flatulent dyspepsia. Combined with antacids in several preparations such as *Asilone*.

Alginates
Dose 1–3 tablets chewed as required.

Protects the mucosa and reduces the incidence of gastro-oesophageal reflux, by floating on the surface of gastric contents. Contained in several preparations such as *Gastro-cote* and *Gaviscon*. Effective in oesophagitis, but dimethicone preparations should not be given concurrently, since they break up the alginate layer.

Anticholinergics
Anticholinergic drugs used in the treatment of peptic ulceration exert their effects by

(*a*) acetylcholine antagonism, reducing gastric acid secretion
(*b*) relaxing smooth muscle, reducing muscle tone and motility and delaying stomach emptying.

Although they may relieve the pain and discomfort in duodenal ulcer, their value in the treatment of ulcers is limited. They are perhaps more useful in motility dysfunction in the gastro-intestinal tract.

Adverse effects. Dry mouth, constipation, urinary retention, impaired vision (Chapter 9).

Hyoscine butylbromide (*Buscopan*)
Dose 10–20 mg orally.

Propantheline bromide (*Pro-Banthine*)
Dose 30 mg at night.
 Useful in relieving duodenal ulcer pain at night.

ANTIDIARRHOEAL DRUGS

Most antidiarrhoeal drugs will relieve the symptoms of diarrhoea without treating the cause. They act by affecting intestinal motility or by absorbing excess water from the gut, thus making the faeces more solid.

Chalk B.P. (calcium carbonate)
Dose 1–5 g orally.

Kaolin
Dose 15 g orally.
 Kaolin is derived from clay and is used to give bulk to faeces. It may be taken as a powder, mixed with a little water or milk or may be incorporated into a mixture.

Opium
Reduces the motility of the intestine and is used in various forms to check diarrhoea.

Chalk and opium mixture
Dose 10–20 ml. orally.

Kaolin and morphine mixture
Dose 10 ml. orally.

Codeine phosphate
Dose 30–60 mg three times a day in tablet or syrup form.

Diphenoxylate
Related to pethidine. Available with small amounts of atropine as *Lomotil*, 1–2 tablets three to four times a day.

Loperamide (*Imodium*)
Dose 2–4 mg.
  A non-absorbable opiate.

  Anticholinergic drugs may, by affecting intestinal motility, relieve diarrhoea and associated colicky pain.

ANTISPASMODICS

Antispasmodics reduce intestinal spasm, and are useful in irritable bowel syndrome.

Dicyclomine hydrochloride (*Debendox, Merbentyl*)
Dose 10 mg three times a day. Available in tablet or syrup form.

Mebeverine (*Colofac*)
Dose 100 mg four times a day.

APERIENTS

Aperients are drugs used in the treatment of constipation. Insufficient vegetable fibre in the diet of western countries has been suggested as one of the major causes of constipation, as well as haemorrhoids, diverticular disease of the colon, irritable bowel syndrome and cancer of the colon. Since bowel habits vary from person to person, so will their criteria of what constitutes constipation. Constipation can be defined as the infrequent, difficult passage of hard stools.
  Many cases of constipation are hospital-induced, where the patient's normal habits are disrupted, due to factors such

as lack of activity, embarrassment, lack of privacy or incorrect position (bedpans). Over-use of aperients can inhibit normal bowel rhythm and induce dependence on the aperients. Often the remedy lies in simple measures such as increasing fluid intake or the use of a proper toilet as opposed to bedpan or commode.

Temporary illness, operations or parturition provide justification for the use of an aperient, as does the necessity to alleviate discomfort in minor rectal operations such as anal fissure and haemorrhoids. Aperients tend to exert their effects in two ways:

(*a*) increase intestinal motility
(*b*) increase water and bulk content of faeces.

Bulk substances

The use of bulk substances is the physiological way of dealing with constipation by increasing the content of the bowel and stimulating peristalsis. They are useful also in solidifying the stool when there is a colostomy or ileostomy.

Bran (*Fybranta*)
Can be taken as natural bran or proprietary preparations.

Ispaghula (*Fybogel, Isogel, Metamucil*)
Dose 5 ml. three times daily.
Derived from plant seed husks.

Sterculia (*Normacol*)
Dose 5–10 g dry on the tongue and swallowed with water.

Methylcellulose (*Celevac*)
Derived from cellulose. When wet, swells and increases the bulk in the intestine.

Saline group

The saline group of drugs exerts an osmotic effect in the colon.

Magnesium sulphate

Dose 5–15 g orally.

Can be also given per rectum to reduce intracranial pressure by the same means.

Magnesium hydroxide (*Milk of magnesia*)

Dose 25–50 ml.

Less potent aperient than magnesium sulphate. It is used also for its antacid properties.

Lactulose (*Duphalac*)

Dose 10 ml.

A non-absorbable disaccharide. Discourages ammonia-producing organisms in the gut; therefore, also used in hepatic encephalopathy.

Lubricants

Lubricants soften the stool and lubricate the intestine and colon, making passage of the stool easier.

Liquid paraffin

Dose 10–30 ml. orally.

Liquid paraffin is a mineral oil obtained from petroleum. The oil tends to separate from the faeces in the rectum and can seep, causing soiling of the clothes. It can also interfere with the absorption of fat soluble vitamins.

Anthracene group

The anthracene group of irritant purgatives are all of vegetable origin and act by stimulating peristalsis 6–8 hours after administration, and so are often given at night. They are not recommended for long-term use. They include senna, cascara, rhubarb and aloes.

Cascara
Dose 2–5 ml. or in tablet form.
   It is prepared from the dried bark of the Sagrada tree and is available as a liquid extract.

Senna
Dose 1–2 tablets, or 1–2 teaspoonfuls of granules.
   Senna is prepared from the leaf and pods of the senna plant. Used in its proprietary brand as *Senokot*.

Castor oil
It is prepared from the seeds of the *Ricinus communis*. It causes drastic purging owing to its irritant effect on the intestine.

Synthetic aperients

Phenolphthalein
Dose 50–200 mg orally.
   Is found in many proprietary preparations and acts by stimulating the large intestine. It is absorbed and re-excreted in the bile, thus giving a repetitive action.

Bisacodyl (*Dulcolax*)
Dose 5–10 mg orally, 10 mg rectally.
   Has a similar action to phenolphthalein. It can also be given as a suppository.

Danthron (*Dorbanex*)
Dose 25–150 mg.
   Stimulates peristalsis. It is a synthetic compound derived from anthracene.

SUPPOSITORIES

Suppositories are drugs prepared for insertion into the rectum. They are usually cone-shaped and are prepared in a base of gelatin or cacao butter, two substances which melt at body temperature. Their chief use is to produce an evacuation of the bowel and to soothe painful mucosa in anal fissure and haemorrhoids.

Suppositories used to produce defaecation

Bisacodyl suppositories (*Dulcolax*)
Dose 10–20 mg.
   Acts by irritating the rectum and colon.

Beogex suppositories
When moist liberate carbon dioxide causing rectal distention and peristalsis.

Glycerol suppositories
Contain glycerine and gelatine, and melt inside rectum providing lubrication.

Suppositories used to soothe mucosa

Anusol suppositories
Proprietary preparation, said to coat the mucous membrane of the rectum.

Suppositories for systemic absorption
Many other drugs which have a systemic action can be given in suppository form, e.g. aminophylline, diazepam, indomethacin.

ANTIEMETICS

Antiemetics are drugs which reduce nausea and vomiting by depressing the vomiting centre in the brain. They are used in travel sickness, pregnancy, uraemia, radiation sickness and patients on cytotoxic drugs.

Hyoscine (*Buscopan*)
Dose 300–600 micrograms.
  The most effective drug in travel sickness.

Phenothiazines
Phenothiazines are potent antiemetics. They also have an antihistamine effect. Their sedative effects, however, mean they should be used with caution if driving or machinery are involved.

Chlorpromazine (*Largactil*)
Dose 25–100 mg orally or by injection.

Promazine (*Sparine*)
Dose 25–100 mg orally or intramuscularly.

Promethazine (*Phenergan*)
Dose 25 mg orally.
  Has stronger antihistamine effects than other phenothiazines. Useful in travel sickness and safe to use in pregnancy.

Perphenazine (*Fentazin*)
Dose 4 mg three times daily orally or intramuscularly.

Prochlorperazine (*Stemetil*)
Dose 5 mg orally.
  Useful in treating vomiting and vertigo in Ménière's disease.

Antihistamines

Most antihistamines have an antiemetic action and are useful in travel sickness and Ménière's disease. However, they also cause drowsiness.

Betahistine (*Serc*)
Dose 8 mg three times daily.

Cinnarizine (*Stugeron*)
Dose 15 mg three times daily.

Cyclizine (*Marzine, Valoid*)
Dose 50 mg four-hourly, tablets or injection.

Dimenhydrinate (*Dramamine*)
Dose 50–100 mg four-hourly, or 50 mg by injection.

Diphenhydramine (*Benadryl*)
Dose 20 mg three times daily.

Metoclopramide (*Maxolon*)
Dose 10 mg orally or by injection.
  Metoclopramide increases peristalsis, so causing quicker gastric emptying. It is also useful in relieving dyspepsia, flatulence and heartburn.

Adverse effects. Extrapyramidal symptoms often of the dystonic type.

DRUGS USED FOR INFLAMMATORY BOWEL DISEASE

Acute cases of Crohn's disease and ulcerative colitis are usually treated with corticosteroids; if the disease is localized to the colon or rectum, enemas or suppositories, respectively, are used to reduce the severity of side-effects due to systemic corticosteroids. Prednisolone is the oral corticosteroid usually given. (See Chapter 13.)

Prednisolone enema (*Predenema, Predsol*)
Dose 1 enema at bedtime.

Care should be taken that patients are administering their own enemas successfully, and can retain them for at least one hour, by lying in the left lateral or prone position.

Prednisolone suppository (*Predsol*)
Dose 1 night and morning and after defaecation.

Hydrocortisone enema (*Cortenema*)
Dose: As for prednisolone enemata. Hydrocortisone suppositories are also available.

Colifoam is a hydrocortisone foam preparation, which reaches most of the colon, and many patients find it easier to use.

Sulphasalazine (*Salazopyrin*)
Dose gradually increased to 2–4 g daily orally.

Sulphasalazine is largely unabsorbed, but is split by bacteria in the colon, into sulphapyridine, which is absorbed, and 5-aminosalicylate, which is the active component, and is not absorbed. It is used to maintain remission in ulcerative colitis, but is less beneficial during an acute attack, than corticosteroids. Although sometimes used in Crohn's disease, its value is uncertain.

MISCELLANEOUS DRUGS

Pancreatin (*Cotazym, Nutrizym, Pancrex, Protopan*)
Dose 2–8 g daily immediately prior to, or sprinkled over, food. Dose adjusted to control steatorrhoea.

These preparations contain pancreatic enzymes, needed

to digest starch, fat and protein. They are given to patients with impaired secretion of these enzymes, due to cystic fibrosis, chronic pancreatitis, or following pancreatectomy, to control malabsorption and steatorrhoea.

Chenodeoxycholic acid (*Chendol, Chenofalk*)
Dose 10–15 mg/kg in divided doses orally for two years.

Chenodeoxycholic acid alters bile composition, so that certain gallstones will eventually dissolve. However, many patients are unsuitable and will still require operation. Ursodeoxycholic acid (*Destolit*), with or without *Rowachol*, promises to be more effective.

Cholestyramine (*Questran*)
Dose 12–24 gm daily orally.

Following small bowel secretion, and certain other diseases, bile salts are not reabsorbed, and can cause diarrhoea by an action in the colon. They are bound by cholestyramine, which is effective treatment for this type of diarrhoea. Also, by preventing cholesterol reabsorption, cholestyramine reduces plasma cholesterol concentration in patients with hypercholesterolaemia (a condition which predisposes to atherosclerosis). Unfortunately, many drugs, such as warfarin, also bind to cholestyramine, and their absorption may be impaired. Vitamin A and D absorption is also affected.

5 Drugs Affecting the Cardiovascular System

DRUGS USED IN CARDIAC FAILURE

Cardiac glycosides

There are many cardiac glycosides produced from the dried leaves of *Digitalis purpura* (digitalis, digitoxin) and *Digitalis lanata* (digoxin). They have been used for many centuries in the treatment of dropsy (oedema). They will improve the work done by the heart without increasing oxygen consumption.

In congestive cardiac failure, they have the following effects:

(*a*) increase the force of myocardial contraction
(*b*) slow the heart by direct depression of the conduction system and by stimulation of the vagus nerve.

These effects will produce relief of respiratory symptoms and a diuresis with relief of oedema. Normal heart rate will be restored in atrial fibrillation and atrial flutter. Different individuals respond differently to the same dose of these drugs, so regular monitoring of serum levels is useful.

Digitalis
Now rarely used.

Digoxin (*Lanoxin*)
The most common glycoside in use. Unless urgent treatment is required, digitalization can be achieved by oral administration, although the dose will vary. Normally an initial

dose of 1 mg in divided doses on the first day, followed by 125–500 micrograms daily will be sufficient to reach therapeutic serum levels. Can also be given intravenously.

Digitoxin (*Digitaline*)
Dose 50–200 micrograms daily. Can also be given intravenously.
   Has a longer half life than digoxin and is more slowly excreted. It is normally given in a lower dosage than digoxin.

Lanatoside C (*Cedilanid*)
Dose 1–1.5 mg daily until digitalization is reached, then 250–270 micrograms daily orally.
   Similar in action to digoxin.

Adverse effects. The margin between the therapeutic and toxic effects is narrow in digitalis preparations. The long half life means that if it is given in repeated doses, then cumulative effects can occur. Early symptoms of overdose include anorexia, nausea and vomiting. A pulse rate of below 60 is also evidence of toxicity and any further administration of the drug should stop. Increased toxicity will cause diarrhoea, abdominal pain, headache, blurred vision, disturbance in colour vision, confusion, and coupling of the pulse. Disturbance in cardiac rhythm is evidence of severe toxicity. Toxic symptoms are more likely to occur in patients concurrently receiving diuretics, where the potassium level is low, and in the elderly. Reduced doses must be given where renal impairment is evident and in the elderly.

Other drugs used in cardiac failure

Diuretics (Chapter 7)
If a patient is in sinus rhythm, diuretics alone are often sufficient to control cardiac failure. If cardiac failure is associated with atrial fibrillation, digoxin is usually preferred, and diuretics added when necessary.

Vasodilators (see pp. 40–41)
Certain vasodilators have recently proved useful in the
treatment of cardiac failure, by reducing cardiac work, and
increasing peripheral blood flow. Such drugs include hydral-
lazine, prazosin, glyceryl trinitrate and captopril.

DRUGS USED IN CARDIAC ARRHYTHMIAS

Quinidine bisulphate (*Kinidin*)
Dose 200–300 mg, three or four times daily orally.
  Quinidine is closely related to quinine. They are both
alkaloids of cinchona bark. Quinidine depresses the excitability of cardiac muscle, slows conduction and prolongs the
refractory period. Quinidine is particularly used in the
treatment of supraventricular arrhythmias, such as parox-
ysmal atrial tachycardia and atrial fibrillation.

Adverse effects. Include cinchonism (i.e. vertigo, tinnitus,
deafness), headache, nausea and vomiting, confusion, skin
rashes and angioedema.

Procainamide (*Pronestyl*)
Dose 0.5–1.5 g orally four-hourly, 25–50 mg intravenously
every 1 min up to 1 g under ECG control.
  Similar in action to quinidine but does not cause cinchonism.
Mainly used for ventricular arrhythmias.

Adverse effects. Hypotension, anorexia, nausea, vomiting,
diarrhoea, weakness, depression, confusion and hallucinations.

Lignocaine (*Lidocaine, Xylocaine*)
Lignocaine is a local anaesthetic used for ventricular arrhythmias. It is often used when ventricular fibrillation
complicates myocardial infarction. With a rapid but short
duration of action, it can be given as a single intravenous
bolus injection of 100 mg, followed by an intravenous

infusion of 1–4 mg/min. It is ineffective when taken orally.
Available as Xylocard preloaded syringes containing 20 mg/ml. and 200 mg/ml.

Adverse effects. Hypotension, drowsiness, muscle twitching, disorientation and convulsions. Lignocaine should not be used in third-degree atrio-ventricular block.

Tocainide is similar to lignocaine, but is also effective when given orally.

Phenytoin (*Epanutin, Dilantin*)
Dose 250 mg by intravenous injection over 5 min: 200–400 mg orally daily.

Related to the barbiturates and a potent anticonvulsant. It is occasionally used in the treatment of ventricular arrhythmias.

Adverse effects. Drowsiness and confusion.

Mexiletine (*Mexitil*)
Dose 600–800 mg daily in divided doses. Can also be given by slow intravenous infusion.

Has a similar effect to lignocaine. Used in ventricular arrhythmias following myocardial infarction and in digitalis toxicity.

Adverse effects. Nausea, confusion, tremor, bradycardia and hypotension. *Contraindicated* in heart block and bradycardia.

Verapamil (*Cordilox*)
Dose 5 mg by slow intravenous injection. Repeat after 10 min if necessary. 120–240 mg orally in divided doses.

Acts by preventing calcium accumulation in myocardial cells. Used in the treatment of atrial arrhythmias.

Adverse effects. Hypotension and bradycardia. *Contra-indicated* in heart block, cardiac failure and bradycardia.

Disopyramide (*Rhythmodan, Norpace*)
Dose by intravenous injection 2 mg/kg body weight to a maximum of 150 mg. Orally 300 mg initially followed by 100 mg four- to six-hourly orally.

Similar in action to quinidine. Used in supraventricular and ventricular arrhythmias.

Adverse effects. Cholinergic-like effects, with dry mouth, retention of urine, blurred vision and constipation.

Amiodarone (*Cordarone X*)
Dose 200 mg one to three times daily.

Very effective treatment for atrial and ventricular arrhythmias, by reducing the excitability of cardiac muscle and conducting tissue. Very slow onset of action, requiring several weeks for maximal effect.

Adverse effects. Corneal deposits, photosensitization and thyroid dysfunction.

Other drugs
These include atropine, digoxin and beta-adrenergic blockers.

BETA ADRENERGIC RECEPTOR BLOCKING DRUGS

Beta blockers are drugs that block sympathetic stimulation of beta receptors in cardiac and smooth muscle. Some beta blockers are selective in action, affecting only cardiac muscle (cardioselective) whilst others affect the myocardium plus smooth muscle in the bronchi and blood vessels (non-selective).

Effects on the heart
Beta blockers have the following effects:

1. Slow the heart rate
2. Reduce myocardial oxygen consumption
3. Lower systemic blood pressure
4. Reduce cardiac output

Therapeutic uses. Beta blockers are useful in preventing attacks of angina during exercise. They also control supraventricular tachycardia, digitalis-induced cardiac irregularities, tachycardia associated with thyrotoxicosis, and hypertension. Their effect in reducing high blood pressure is probably due more to their action on the vasomotor centre in the brain, but they may also have an anti-renin effect.

Adverse effects. Beta blockers may precipitate cardiac failure and bronchospasm, nausea, diarrhoea, insomnia, hallucinations and depression. They are *contraindicated* in patients in heartblock, cardiac failure and those with a history of asthma or bronchospasm. Patients with peripheral vascular disease should be given cardioselective beta blockers only.

Propranolol hydrochloride (*Inderal, Berkolol*)
Dose 30 mg–320 mg daily orally, 500 micrograms–1 mg by intravenous injection.
   Propranolol is a non-selective beta blocker, used in the treatment of angina, hypertension, cardiac arrhythmias and thyrotoxicosis. It can also be used to control the somatic features of anxiety.

Oxprenolol hydrochloride (*Trasicor*)
Dose 40–480 mg daily in divided doses, 1–2 mg by slow intravenous injection.

Timolol maleate (*Blocadren, Betim*)
Dose 15–45 mg daily in divided doses.

Sotalol hydrochloride (*Beta-cardone, Sotacor*)
Dose 120–480 mg daily in divided doses.

Pindolol (*Visken*)
Dose 10–45 mg daily in divided doses.

Cardioselective beta blockers

Practolol (*Eraldin*)
Dose 5 mg by slow intravenous injection, repeat after 5 min.
   Is available only as an intravenous preparation for acute arrhythmias.

Acebutolol (*Sectral*)
Dose 300–800 mg daily in divided doses.

Atenolol (*Tenormin*)
Dose 100 mg daily.

Metoprolol (*Betaloc, Lopresor*)
Dose 50–400 mg daily in divided doses, 5 mg by intravenous injection.

DRUGS USED IN ANGINA PECTORIS

Nitrates

The nitrates are a group of drugs that act on the smooth muscle of the body causing it to relax. This effect is particularly marked in the arterial walls. Their effectiveness in angina may be due to relieving coronary artery spasm and to the reduction in venous pressure and cardiac output, which places less demand for oxygen on the myocardium. Nitrates are rapidly absorbed from mucous membranes.

Glyceryl trinitrate (*Trinitrine*)
Dose 0.5–1 mg taken sublingually. No more than two tablets should be taken at a time. These tablets are ineffective if swallowed. Sustained-release tablets should be swallowed, 2.6–6.4 mg two or three times daily.

Isosorbide dinitrate (*Vascardin, Sorbitrate, Cedocard, Isordil*)
Dose 5–10 mg sublingually, 5–20 mg two to four times daily.
Used in the treatment and prophylaxis of angina. Similar in action to glyceryl trinitrate.

Pentaerythritol tetranitrate (*Cardiacap, Mycardol, Peritrate*)
Dose 60–180 mg daily in divided doses.
A long-acting nitrate used in the prophylaxis of angina.

Other drugs used to treat angina pectoris

Perhexiline (*Pexid*)
Dose 200–400 mg daily in divided doses.
Used in the prophylaxis of angina. Long-term treatment may produce raised intracranial pressure, peripheral neuropathy and hepatitis.

Nifedipine (*Adalat*)
Dose 30–60 mg daily in divided doses.
Used in the treatment and prophylaxis of angina. Acts by relieving coronary artery spasm and reducing arterial pressure.

Beta receptor blockers
If the nitrates are ineffective in controlling angina or cannot

be tolerated, then one of the beta blocker drugs may be given. Their effects on the heart have been discussed earlier. The possibility of precipitating cardiac failure, however, should be borne in mind.

PERIPHERAL VASODILATORS

Peripheral vasodilators are drugs used to improve the circulation by reducing vasospasm in disorders such as Raynaud's disease. They may also be used to improve the collateral circulation in arteriosclerosis or atherosclerosis, but their effectiveness in these disorders is doubtful. Some vasodilators are used in the management of hypertension, cardiac failure and angina pectoris, and are discussed under these headings.

Peripheral vasodilators can act by:

(*a*) Blocking the effect of adrenaline on receptor sites in skin blood vessels, thereby producing vasodilation (alpha adrenergic blocking drugs)
(*b*) Direct effect on the blood vessel wall.

Alpha adrenergic blockers

Tolazoline (*Priscol*)
Used in the treatment of peripheral vascular disease.

Adverse effects. Increases gastric acid secretion and causes diarrhoea and tachycardia. A *contraindication* is peptic ulcer.

Phenoxybenzamine (*Dibenyline*)
Dose 80 mg three times daily orally. Can also be used intravenously.

Has a more prolonged action than tolazoline. Used before

and during surgery for phaeochromocytoma and for Raynaud's disease.

Adverse effects. Postural hypotension, tachycardia, nausea and vomiting.

Phentolamine (*Rogitine*)
Dose 5–10 mg intravenously. Can be repeated.
   A short-acting mild alpha blocker, used mainly in the treatment of phaeochromocytoma. Can also be used in the hypertensive crisis due to the interaction between monoamine oxidase inhibitors and tyramine-containing foods.

Adverse effects. As for phenoxybenzamine.

Drugs which have a direct action on the blood vessel wall

Thymoxamine (*Opilon*)
Dose 40 mg four times daily. Can also be used intravenously.
   Used in the treatment of peripheral vascular disorders.

Adverse effects. Nausea, diarrhoea, headache, flushing.

Bamethan sulphate (*Vasculit*)
Used in the treatment of Raynaud's disease.

Adverse effects. Postural hypotension, tachycardia. A *contra-indication* is recent myocardial infarction.

Nicotinic acid derivatives. Used in the treatment of chilblains and frostbite.

Nicotinic acid (*Ronicol*)
Dose 25–50 mg four times daily orally.

Inositol nicotinate (*Hexopal*)
Dose 1.5–3 g daily.

Nicofuranose (*Bradilan*)
Dose 500 mg three times daily.

Cyclandelate (*Cyclospasmol*)
Dose 1.2–1.6 g daily in divided doses.

Adverse effects. Flushing, dizziness.

Co-dergocrine mesylate (*Hydergine*)
Used mainly to improve cerebral blood flow in senile dementia.

Adverse effects. Nausea, vomiting, flushing, postural hypotension.

Isoxsuprine (*Duvadilan*)
Dose 20 mg four times daily. Can also be given parenterally.

DRUGS USED IN THE TREATMENT OF HYPERTENSION

It is difficult to decide at which point a raised blood pressure can be considered hypertensive. The majority of people with raised blood pressure do not suffer symptoms; therefore energetic treatment with drugs which might produce severe adverse effects might be counterproductive. It is generally thought, however, that a persistent raised diastolic pressure of above 100 mm Hg, requires active treatment to prevent the often fatal consequences of a severe myocardial infarction, cardiac and renal failure. Investigations should be undertaken to determine whether the raised blood pressure is secondary to existing disorders such as phaeochromocytoma. In the majority of hypertensive patients, however, no existing cause can be found. The main factors responsible for the maintenance of blood pressure within normal limits include cardiac output and peripheral resistance. Most of the anti-hypertensive drugs affect the peripheral resistance in a variety of different ways.

Thiazide diuretics and **beta blockers** are drugs of first choice in controlling mild and moderate hypertension and can be used in combination. **Labetalol hydrochloride** (*Trandate*) is useful with both alpha and beta blocker effects. Other drugs may be added if control remains unsatisfactory.

Vasodilator Drugs

These reduce peripheral resistance by relaxing the smooth muscle walls of the arteries.

Hydrallazine (*Apresoline*)

Dose to control severe hypertension, 10–20 mg by slow intravenous injection. Orally 75–200 mg daily in divided doses.

Particularly useful when combined with beta blockers. Used in the treatment of moderate to severe hypertension, and cardiac failure.

Adverse effects. Tachycardia, hypotension, flushing, nasal congestion. Chronic administration can cause a systemic lupus erythematosus-like syndrome.

Diazoxide (*Eudemine*)

Dose 300 mg given intravenously.

Only used in hypertensive crisis and is not suitable for regular use.

Adverse effects. Tachycardia, hyperglycaemia, fluid retention.

Sodium nitroprusside (*Nipride***)**
Dose 0.5–1.5 micrograms/kg body weight initially. Infusion solution must be protected from light.
  Used in the treatment of hypertensive crisis.

Adverse effects. Headache, vomiting, dizziness. *Contra-indications* are renal and hepatic failure.

Prazosin (*Hypovase***)**
Dose 0.5 mg three times daily increasing to a maximum dose of 20 mg daily.

Adverse effects. Loss of consciousness, postural hypotension.

Captopril (*Capoten***)**
Dose initially 25 mg three times daily.
  Acts by interfering with the renin-angiotension system and is effective in severe hypertension and cardiac failure.

Adverse effects. Loss of taste, rashes, proteinuria, renal failure, blood dyscrasias, hyperkalaemia.

Minoxidil (*Loniten***)**
Dose 5–50 mg daily orally.
  The most powerful vasodilator.

Adverse effects. Marked fluid retention—diuretics should always be given. Tachycardia, which can be prevented by beta blockers. Hirsutism.

Centrally acting drugs

This group of drugs have a direct action on the hypothalamus and on the peripheral sympathetic nerves. The anti-hypertensive effect may result from either action.

Rauwolfia (Reserpine) (*Serpasil*)
Dose 250–500 micrograms orally daily.

Acts by depleting central and peripheral stores of nor-adrenaline. Its central action produces a calming effect but can also cause severe depression with an increased risk of suicide.

Adverse effects. Bradycardia, postural hypotension, nasal congestion, sedation, fluid retention and Parkinsonian-like effects. *Contraindications* include patients with a history of depression or Parkinson's disease.

Clonidine (*Catapres*)
Dose 0.05–0.1 mg three times daily, increasing the dose every third day, until control of hypertension is reached.

This drug must never be stopped abruptly as that may precipitate a hypertensive crisis.

Adverse effects. Sedation, dry mouth, depression and Raynaud's phenomenon.

Methyldopa (*Aldomet*)
Dose 250 mg three times daily, gradually increasing to a maximum dose of 3 g daily. Can be used intravenously in hypertensive crisis.

Has both central and peripheral action. It is often combined with a diuretic for more effective results.

Adverse effects. Depression, drowsiness, sedation, fluid retention, vomiting, diarrhoea, nasal congestion, liver damage, haemolytic anaemia. *Contraindications* include history of depression, liver disease and phaeochromocytoma.

Ganglion blocking drugs
These act by blocking the effect of acetylcholine at autonomic

ganglia, thus preventing constriction of blood vessels. They affect, however, both sympathetic and para-sympathetic ganglia, producing anticholinergic side effects. Because of this, they are rarely used. Drugs contained in this group include pentolinium (*Ansolysen*), mecamylamine (*Inversine*) and pempidine (*Tenormal*).

Post-ganglionic blocking drugs

By blocking the release of noradrenaline at sympathetic nerve endings only, these drugs produce a vasodilation in arterioles and consequent lowering of blood pressure without producing anticholinergic side effects.

Guanethidine (*Ismelin*)

Dose 10 mg daily increasing by 10 mg every few days.

Adverse effects. Postural hypotension, severe diarrhoea, vomiting, impotence.

Bethanidine (*Esbatal*)

Dose 10 mg three times daily increasing by 5 mg every two days.

Action similar to that of guanethidine, although shorter acting. This means that the dosage can be increased more rapidly.

Adverse effects. As guanethidine.

Debrisoquine sulphate (*Declinax*)

Dose 10 mg twice daily increasing by 10 mg every three days.

Has fewer adverse effects than other drugs in this group. Often given with thiazide diuretics.

Guanoclor sulphate (*Vatensol*)
Dose 5 mg twice daily.

Guanoxon (*Envacar*)

VASOCONSTRICTORS

The vasoconstrictors are preparations which raise the blood pressure by their action on the peripheral blood vessels. They have been used in the past in emergencies where hypotension was marked, as after myocardial infarction or surgical shock. Their use is not now recommended because of their effect in reducing the perfusion of blood to other vital organs.

Metaraminol tartrate (*Aramine*)
Dose 2–10 mg by intramuscular or subcutaneous injection, 15–100 mg intravenously in 500 ml. sodium chloride.

Methoxamine (*Vasoxine*)
Dose 5–20 mg intravenously or intramuscularly.
   Useful in hypotension occurring during anaesthesia.

Noradrenaline acid tartrate
Dose 2–20 micrograms/min by slow intravenous infusion.

DRUGS AFFECTING CLOT FORMATION

Anticoagulants
Anticoagulants are substances which are given to interfere with the clotting of blood. The formation of clots within blood vessels is a complex matter involving many factors. The end result is the conversion of fibrinogen to insoluble fibrin by the action of thrombin. Fibrin forms a mesh trapping platelets and red blood cells, forming a clot. Calcium ions and vitamin

K are among the substances essential for the clotting process. Thrombin formation can occur in both arteries and veins. In arteries platelets play the important role, while in veins fibrin is more important.

Anticoagulants are of little value in preventing thrombin formation in the faster flowing blood in arteries. Their main use is in the prevention and treatment of deep venous thrombosis, and thrombi in the cardiac chamber, as may occur, for example, in mitral stenosis.

Deep vein thrombosis can arise under a variety of conditions:

1. When the blood is not flowing adequately (stasis) such as may arise in prolonged bed rest.
2. Where the person has a tendency to clot formation or has a defective clot dissolving system.

Females during pregnancy or who are taking a contraceptive pill also have an increased tendency to clot formation.

Heparin

Heparin is given by intravenous injection 5000–10 000 units six-hourly or by continuous infusion of 40 000 units over 24 hours. It can also be given prior to surgery, 5000 units subcutaneously, the day prior to surgery and thereafter at 12-hourly intervals until discharge. If continuous intravenous administration is undertaken, then it is advisable to monitor the blood clotting time and thrombin time.

Heparin is a naturally occurring substance produced by the liver. It inhibits the formation of thrombin from pro-thrombin. It is not absorbed when taken orally so must be given by injection. Heparin is also painful to administer intramuscularly but can be given subcutaneously. It is usual, however, to administer by intravenous injection. It has a rapid onset of action but short duration of effect, so must be given at least six-hourly.

Therapeutic uses. Heparin is often administered at the beginning of anticoagulant therapy until oral anticoagulants take effect. Its main value following a coronary thrombosis may lie in the prevention of deep venous thrombosis. Heparin is often given to patients prior to open-heart surgery and in haemodialysis. In low doses it can be given to prevent post-operative deep vein thrombosis and pulmonary embolus.

Adverse effects. Heparin in large doses may cause bleeding, and haematuria may be the first sign that this has occurred. Treatment is to withdraw the heparin. If bleeding is severe, protamine sulphate (1 mg for every 100 units of heparin given) will reverse the effects of heparin. *Contraindications* include patients with peptic ulcer, haemophilia and severe hypertension.

Oral anticoagulants

Oral anticoagulants act by interfering with the formation of vitamin K dependent coagulation factors, which increases the prothrombin time. Because of their slow onset of action, they are often combined with heparin initially in treatment. Blood prothrombin time should be monitored and dosage adjusted accordingly. They are used in the treatment of deep venous thrombosis and in patients with atrial fibrillation to prevent emboli formation. They may also be effective in preventing transient cerebral ischaemic attacks.

Warfarin (*Warfarin, Marevan*)
Dose initially 20–30 mg orally on the first day of treatment, followed by 10 mg on the second day and thereafter 3–10 mg daily.

Phenindione (*Dindevan*)
Dose 200–300 mg as an initial dose followed by 100 mg on the second day and thereafter 25–100 mg daily.

Nicoumalone (*Sinthrome*)
Dose 8–16 mg on the first day followed by 4–12 mg on the second day. Maintenance dose usually 1–6 mg daily.

Fibrinolytic drugs

Fibrin is formed as part of the normal clotting process, whenever there is damage to the vascular tree. However, it is likely that fibrin is constantly being formed and dissolved in the plasma. Plasminogen is an inert gamma globulin present in blood, which, when activated, is converted to plasmin, which dissolves fibrin. The enzyme necessary for this activation is normally found in blood, urine and in large quantities in damaged tissues.

Fibrinolytic drugs activate plasminogen to form plasmin.

Streptokinase (*Streptase, Kabikinase*)
Dose 500 000 units administered intravenously over 30 min initially, followed by 100 000 units hourly by intravenous infusion for 5–7 days.

Obtained from certain strains of streptococci. It is used in the treatment of thromboembolic disorders such as deep venous thrombosis and pulmonary embolus.

Adverse effects. Pyrexia, anaphylaxis. Haemorrhage is a danger, so careful monitoring of thrombin time is essential.

Urokinase
Dose intraocular administration 5000 units in 2 ml. sodium chloride.

A naturally occurring substance found in urine, used for its thrombolytic effect in eye disorders and for cleaning arterio-venous shunts.

Adverse effects. Similar to streptokinase.

Antifibrinolytic drugs

These are substances that inhibit the activation of plasminogen and therefore prevent the breakdown of fibrin and clots.

Aminocaproic acid (*Epsikapron*)
Dose 3 g four to six times daily.

Used to reverse the action of streptokinase, and in the treatment of severe haemorrhage following prostatectomy, and in subarachnoid haemorrhage.

Adverse effects. Nausea and diarrhoea.

Tranexamic acid (*Cyklokapron*)
Dose by slow intravenous injection 1–20 g three times daily. Orally 1 g three or four times daily.

Aprotinin (*Trasylol*)
A polypeptide which inhibits both plasmin and trypsin. Used in the treatment of haemorrhage associated with fibrinolysis. Its value in the treatment of pancreatitis is questionable.

Antiplatelet drugs

These are drugs that inhibit platelets adhering to each other, and so prevent thrombin formation, particularly in arteries, where platelet aggregation is pronounced. Aspirin has this effect and is known to prolong the bleeding time. Its therapeutic usefulness in preventing arterial thrombus formation, however, has not been established.

Dipyridamole (*Persantin*)
Dose 100–200 mg four times daily.

It can be used to prevent thrombus development in prosthetic values in conjunction with anticoagulants.

Adverse effects. Nausea, diarrhoea, hypotension.

Sulphinpyrazone (*Anturan*)
Dose 200 mg four times daily.
May be of value in patients following a myocardial infarction.

SCLEROSING AGENTS

These agents are substances which, when injected into veins, cause an inflammatory process and the formation of a sterile blood clot. They are used in the treatment of varicose veins and haemorrhoids.

Varicose veins

Ethanolamine oleate
Dose 2–5 ml. injection in separate sites.
Should be used with caution as extravasation will cause tissue necrosis.

Haemorrhoids

Phenol in oil
Dose 0.5–1.5 ml.
Contains 5% phenol in almond/olive oil which is injected into the submucous layer around the haemorrhoid.

DRUGS USED IN THE TREATMENT OF HYPERLIPIDAEMIA

The elevation of blood lipids is thought to be one of the risk factors associated with coronary artery disease. A diet low in animal or saturated fats but high in vegetable or polyunsaturated fats may help to reduce blood lipid levels.

Drugs given to reduce blood lipids usually interfere with cholesterol or triglycerides formation. There is no conclusive evidence that reduction in dietary fats or administration of drugs prevent the onset of myocardial infarction.

Cholestyramine (*Questran*)
Dose 12–16 g daily in divided doses.
  Prevents absorption of cholesterol from the intestine.

Colestipol (*Colestid*)
Dose 15–20 g daily in divided doses.
  Similar in action to cholestyramine.

Clofibrate (*Atromid-S*)
Dose 1–2 g daily.
  Lowers blood triglyceride levels as well as cholesterol.

Adverse effects. Gastric upsets, increases gall-stone formation and myopathy.

6 Drugs Affecting the Respiratory System

These include all preparations which act on any structure from the nose to the lungs.

INHALATIONS

These preparations, when added to nearly boiling water, are inhaled, and have a soothing effect on upper respiratory tract inflammation. However, the symptomatic relief is largely due to humidification from steam rather than the additive.

Benzoin and menthol inhalations
Dose 5 ml. in 600 ml. at 70°C.

EXPECTORANTS

Although used to stimulate coughing, they are clinically ineffective.

MUCOLYTICS

These reduce the viscosity of sputum to aid expectoration, but are probably clinically ineffective. However, adequate humidification and maintenance of an adequate fluid balance are of major importance.

Acetylcysteine (*Airbron*)
Dose 2–5 ml. of a 20% solution as a nebulized inhalation.

Bromhexine (*Bisolvon*)
Dose 8–16 mg four times daily orally.

COUGH SUPPRESSANTS

These are opiates which depress the cough centre in the medulla oblongata. However, they may also seriously depress respiration. Also, since a productive cough should never be suppressed, cough suppressants are rarely indicated, except for:

1. Troublesome nocturnal non-productive cough in acute respiratory tract infections.
2. Intractable malignant disease. Large doses of oral opiates may be given if necessary.

Linctus codeine
Dose 15 mg in 5 ml.

Diamorphine linctus
Dose 1.5–6 mg orally.

BRONCHODILATOR DRUGS

These reverse the airways obstruction, which is a feature of asthma. Reversible airways obstruction is sometimes associated with chronic bronchitis.
   They are divided into four groups:

Adrenergic agonists
These act on bronchial beta-2 receptors.

Adrenaline
Dose 0.2 to 0.5 ml. of 1:1000 solution subcutaneously.

However, it also produces vasoconstriction (via alpha-adrenergic receptors) and cardiac stimulation (via beta-1 adrenergic receptors). Adrenaline and other beta-2 agonists, such as isoprenaline and orciprenaline (*Alupent*) have been largely superseded by specific beta-2 agonists, which have minimal alpha and beta-1 agonist activity.

Salbutamol (*Ventolin*)

This is considered the drug of choice in the treatment of bronchial asthma, and is a specific beta-2 agonist (see Table 1).

Other beta-2 agonists similar to salbutamol are: **Terbutaline** *(Bricanyl)*, **Fenoterol** *(Berotec)*, **Isoetharine** *(Numotac)*, **Reproterol** *(Bronchodil)*, and **Rimiterol** *(Pulmadil)*

Table 1. Salbutamol administration

Route	Dose	Comments
Oral	4 mg 6-hourly	Higher doses produce tremor, anxiety and tachycardia. These effects are minimized by inhalation, now the preferred method of administration.
Inhalation		
(*a*) Aerosol	100–200 micrograms 6-hourly	Requires correct use of aerosol for maximum benefit.
(*b*) Rotacaps	400 micrograms 6-hourly	Easier to use than aerosol, especially in very young children.
(*c*) Respirator solution	2 ml. of 0.5% solution over 3 min	Requires little patient co-operation—especially useful in severe asthma. Nebulizer required.

Theophylline

These are used in combination with beta-2 agonists. Unfortunately, no inhaled preparations are available, and usefulness is limited by frequent side effects.

Choline theophyllinate (*Choledyl*)

Sustained-release theophylline (*Phyllocontin Continus*)
Dose 100–400 mg two to four times daily orally.

Adverse effects. Gastric irritation, arrhythmias, cerebral stimulation and convulsions. Aminophylline suppositories are similar (proctitis instead of gastritis!)

Aminophylline
Dose 5 mg/kg over 30 min, then 500 mg eight-hourly by intravenous infusion. Liver dysfunction necessitates reduced dosage.
    Very useful in acute severe asthma.

Adverse effects. Similar to theophylline. Dosage by either route should be adjusted according to plasma theophylline concentrations.

Anticholinergic drugs

Ipratropium (*Atrovent*)
Dose 40 micrograms six-hourly by aerosol.
    Much less effective than beta-2 agonists in younger patients, but may be superior in asthmatic bronchitics, when useful bronchodilation may be produced by combined ipratropium and beta-2 agonists. No significant side effects.

Corticosteroids

Their effectiveness in asthma is probably due to:

1. Supression of allergic reactions.
2. Sensitization of bronchial smooth muscle to beta-2 agonists.

These are the only effective drugs in severe asthma. Steroids are also sometimes used to prevent fibrosis in sarcoidosis and fibrosing alveolitis. The many side effects of corticosteroids are described in Chapter 13.

Prednisolone
Dose 20 mg four times daily orally in acute asthmatic exacerbations, tailing off or reducing the dose as soon as possible. For alternative oral preparations, see Chapter 13.

Hydrocortisone
Dose 200 mg six-hourly intravenously in severe asthma.

Beclomethasone dipropionate (*Becotide*)
Dose 100 micrograms six-hourly by aerosol inhalation.

Betamethasone valerate (*Bextasol*)
Dose 200 micrograms six-hourly by aerosol inhalation.
   Should be taken regularly as a prophylaxis when other drugs are inadequate. The aerosol avoids systemic side-effects of steroids.

INHIBITORS OF HYPERSENSITIVITY REACTIONS

These are used as asthma prophylaxis and prevent the release of mediators, e.g. SRS-A, following exposure to allergens. They must be taken regularly, and are useless during an acute attack. Only effective in younger patients, especially when external allergens precipitate asthma.

Sodium cromoglycate (*Intal*)
Dose inhaled powder 1 capsule six-hourly (not absorbed).

Ketotifen (*Zaditen*)
Dose 1–2 mg once or twice daily.
   Oral asthma prophylactic—not as effective as cromoglycate.

RESPIRATORY STIMULANTS

These directly stimulate the respiratory centre, increasing the rate and depth of respiration. However, even at therapeutic doses, they may cause cerebral stimulation, resulting in excitement and convulsions. *Indications*: Acute or chronic respiratory failure; post anaesthesia.

Doxapram (*Dopram*)
Dose 100 mg intravenously or preferably by infusion.
   This is now the drug of choice, since there is no cerebral stimulation at therapeutic concentrations.

Nikethamide
Dose 500 mg–2 g by slow intravenous infusion.

7 Drugs Acting on the Kidneys

DIURETICS

These are drugs that increase the production of urine by the kidneys. Many substances can exert a diuretic effect either by:

1. Increasing the flow of blood through the kidneys, e.g. xanthine derivatives such as caffeine and the cardiac glycosides such as digoxin.
2. Interfering with the reabsorption of ions in the kidney tubules. It is this group that we shall consider here.

Thiazide group

These act by inhibiting the amount of sodium and chloride reabsorbed from the kidney tubules. This permits an increased renal excretion of water. The increased concentration of sodium in the distal tubules allows potassium to be exchanged for sodium, with the result that potassium is lost in the urine.

Therapeutic uses. The thiazides are effective in relieving oedema caused by congestive cardiac failure, hepatic and renal disease. They also have a hypotensive effect, and are often the first choice drug in the control of hypertension.

Adverse effects. The thiazides have few side effects in low doses. They may cause hyperglycaemia and aggravate diabetes mellitus. They increase blood uric acid levels and may precipitate an attack of gout. Despite the loss of potassium in the urine, potassium supplements are not always necessary. Serum potassium concentrations, however, should be regularly assessed in patients taking thiazides. Skin rashes and thrombocytopaenia occasionally occur. *Contraindications:* renal failure.

Chlorothiazide (*Saluric*)
Dose 500 mg–2 g daily.
    Produces a rapid diuresis within 30 min and has a maximal effect within two–four hours which ceases after 12 hours.

Hydrochlorothiazide (*Hydrosaluric, Esidrex, Direma*)
Dose 25–200 mg daily.

Bendrofluazide (*Neo-Naclex, Berkozide, Aprinox*)
Dose 2.5–10 mg daily.
    Has a longer duration of action than chlorothiazide.

Hydroflumethiazide (*Hydrenox*)
Dose 25–200 mg daily.

Chlorthalidone (*Hygroton*)
Dose 25–100 mg daily or 50–200 mg on alternate days.
    A synthetic preparation which resembles the thiazides and has a longer duration of action.

Clopamide (*Brinaldix*)
Dose 20–60 mg daily.

Cyclopenthiazide (*Navidrex*)
Dose 0.25–1 mg daily.

Polythiazide (*Nephril*)
Dose 1–4 mg daily.

Quinethazone (*Aquamox*)
Dose 50–100 mg daily.

Methyclothiazide (*Enduron*)
Dose 2.5–10 mg daily.

Mefruside (*Baycaron*)
Dose 25–50 mg daily.

Clorexolone (*Nefrolan*)
Dose 20–100 mg daily.

Indapamide (*Natrilix*)
Dose 2.5 mg daily.

Metolazone (*Metenix*)
Dose 5–20 mg daily.
   More potent than other thiazides; effective in renal failure.

Xipamide (*Diurexan*)
Dose 20–40 mg daily.

Loop diuretics

Frusemide (*Lasix, Dryptal, Frusetic, Frusid*)
Dose 20–40 mg once daily orally—for emergency use 20–40 mg intramuscularly or slow intravenously. In renal failure, up to 1 g daily.
   Although related to the thiazides, frusemide is a more powerful and shorter acting diuretic. It acts principally on the ascending limb of the loop of Henle, producing a diuresis within 30 min and lasting up to six hours. Useful where urgent action is required to relieve oedema in cardiac and renal failure.

Adverse effects. The massive diuresis sometimes produced can cause a reduction in blood volume and hypotension. Tinnitus and deafness can occur with high doses, especially

in renal failure. Other side effects are as for thiazides, but
potassium loss may be less, except with higher doses.

Ethacrynic acid (*Edecrin*)
Dose 50–200 mg daily orally, 50 mg by slow intravenous
injection.
   Similar in action to frusemide.

Bumetanide (*Burinex*)
Dose 500 micrograms–2 mg daily. Can also be used
intravenously.
   Related to frusemide. It has a rapid onset but short
duration.

Potassium-sparing diuretics

These are weak diuretics but they also reduce the amount of
potassium excreted in the urine. Consequently, potassium
supplements should not be given with these drugs. They are
most useful when combined with other diuretics, to prevent
potassium depletion.

Spironolactone (*Aldactone A*)
Dose 100–200 mg daily.
   A synthetic steroid which acts by blocking the action of the
salt retaining hormone aldosterone. It is useful in conditions
associated with aldosterone excess such as oedema due to
cirrhosis of the liver, and severe cardiac failure.

Adverse effects. Gynaecomastia, gastro-intestinal upsets
and hyperkalaemia. *Contraindications*: hyperkalaemia, renal
failure.

Triamterene (*Dytac*)
Dose 150–250 mg daily.

Acts by blocking sodium/potassium exchange in the distal tubule and has a weak diuretic effect. Also available combined with thiazide (*Dytide, Dyazide*).

Adverse effects. Skin rashes, confusion, hyperkalaemia. *Contraindications*: hyperkalaemia, anuria, renal disease, pregnancy.

Amiloride (*Midamor*)
Dose 5–10 mg daily.
Similar in action to triamterene. *Moduretic* contains 5 mg amiloride with 50 mg hydrochlorothiazide.

Osmotic diuretics

These drugs exert an osmotic effect in the renal tubules, causing less water to be reabsorbed. Although the diuretic effect is mild, they are useful in reducing cerebral oedema. They must be given intravenously.

Mannitol
Dose 25–200 g daily as a 10, 15 or 20% aqueous solution. *Contraindications*: congestive cardiac failure and pulmonary oedema.

Urea (*Ureaphil*)
Dose 40–80 g as a 30% solution in dextrose.

Mercurial diuretics

Mersalyl
It is rarely used now because of its severe toxic effects.

Adverse effects. Ventricular fibrillation, nausea, vomiting, fever, urticaria, agranulocytosis, renal failure.

POTASSIUM SUPPLEMENTS

These are seldom required with low doses of thiazides or loop diuretics. Reducing excessive salt intake reduces potassium loss, and also the need for higher doses of diuretics. Potassium-retaining diuretics are often more effective at correcting hypokalaemia, and mean less tablets for the patient than potassium supplements.

Potassium bicarbonate
Contains 6.5 mmol potassium in an effervescent tablet. May cause oesophageal and small bowel ulceration.

Potassium chloride
Available as a syrup (*Kay-Cee-L*), effervescent preparations (*Kloref, Sando-K*) or sustained-release preparations (to prevent gastric irritation and gut ulceration; *K-Contin, Leo-K, Slow-K*).

Potassium gluconate (*Katorin*)

Combined diuretic and potassium supplements
These drugs are now less widely used, since they contain insufficient potassium. Examples of these drugs are:

  Lasix + K (40 mg frusemide + potassium)
  Lasikal (20 mg frusemide + potassium)
  Diumide-K (40 mg frusemide + potassium)
  Navidrex-K (0.25 mg cyclopenthiazide + potassium)
  Neo-Naclex-K (2.5 mg bendrofluazide + potassium)
  Brinaldix-K (20 mg clopamide + potassium).

8 Drugs Affecting the Central Nervous System

ANALGESICS

These are drugs given to relieve pain. The experience of pain is a subjective phenomenon influenced by:

1. The degree of noxious stimulus and tissue damage.
2. The individual's awareness and response to the pain.

The latter is influenced by the patient's emotional state, attitudes, previous learning, culture and available distractions. The transmission of painful stimuli within the brain and spinal cord is inhibited by the release of neurotransmitters called enkephalins, and it may be that these attenuating influences act by causing release of enkephalins.

Mild to moderate pain is often musculoskeletal in origin. Many drugs which are successful in producing pain relief in this group also have anti-inflammatory and antipyretic effects. Their site of action is thought to be predominately in the peripheral nerves.

Narcotic analgesics are used for severe pain often originating in the viscera. Their sites of action are the enkephalin receptors in the brain and spinal cord.

Analgesics used for moderate pain

Aspirin (acetylsalicylic acid)
Aspirin belongs to a group of drugs called salicylates which

have antipyretic, anti-inflammatory and analgesic properties. Although aspirin seems to have peripheral and central effects, its exact mode of action in producing analgesia is unknown. It is, however, an effective analgesic in a variety of musculoskeletal pains and headache. Its anti-inflammatory effect is probably due to blockade of prostaglandin synthesis. In large dosage it is often the first drug to be used in rheumatoid arthritis and rheumatic fever. Aspirin also exerts an antipyretic effect when the temperature is raised, by 'resetting' the temperature control centre in the hypothalamus.

Adverse effects. Side effects are generally mild, but may cause gastric irritation and bleeding. Allergic reactions such as skin rashes and asthmatic attacks can occur. Mild intoxication with aspirin causes 'salicylism', characterized by deafness, dizziness, tinnitus, confusion, vomiting and hyperventilation. Severe toxic levels can result in metabolic acidosis and death. *Contraindications*. Aspirin should not be given to individuals with gastric ulceration or those prone to asthmatic attacks. Aspirin and alcohol excess is particularly likely to cause gastritis.

Aspirin tablets
Dose 300–900 mg, four–six hourly.

Soluble aspirin (*Dispirin*)
Dose 300–900 mg, four–six hourly.

Sodium salicylate
Dose 500 mg–1 g, four-hourly.
This is a less effective analgesic than aspirin, and is more likely to cause gastric irritation. Used in the treatment of rheumatic fever.

Aspirin and codeine tablets (compound codeine tablets)
Dose 1–2 tablets.

Contain acetylsalicylic acid 250 mg and codeine phosphate 8 mg.

Calcium aspirin
Dose 1–2 tablets twice daily.

Contains 500 mg aspirin and 150 mg calcium carbonate. Used in the treatment of rheumatic conditions.

Aspirin and caffeine tablets and powders
Used in the treatment of colds, influenza and rheumatic pain.

Paediatric preparations of aspirin are also available. Many proprietary brands of aspirin are often sold combined with other substances.

Aloxiprin (*Palaprin*)
Dose 1–2 tablets orally.

A combination of aluminium oxide and aspirin, which releases the analgesic in the intestine, in an attempt to reduce gastric irritation.

Benorylate (*Benoral*)
Dose 1–1.5 g six-hourly.

This is an aspirin and paracetamol compound.

Paracetamol (*Panadol*)
Dose 500 mg–1 g four times daily.

Paracetamol is a milder analgesic than aspirin and does not have anti-inflammatory properties. However, it does not cause gastric irritation and bleeding.

Adverse effects. In overdosage it can cause liver necrosis.

Mefenamic acid (*Ponstan*)
Dose 500 mg, three times daily.

A stronger analgesic than aspirin, but long-term treatment with this drug is not recommended.

Adverse effects. Gastric irritation, drowsiness, diarrhoea and occasionally blood dyscrasias.

Flufenamic acid (*Meralen*)
Dose 200 mg, three times daily.
   Similar to mefenamic acid.

Carbamazepine (*Tegretol*)
Dose 100–200 mg orally, four times daily.
   A phenothiazine derivative with anticonvulsant properties. Although not strictly an analgesic, carbamazepine is very effective in the treatment of trigeminal neuralgia.

Compound analgesic preparations
There are many other compound analgesic preparations available, including *Distalgesic, Fantagesic, Norgesic, Paramol-118*, some of which contain small doses of opiates. Their advantage over simpler preparations has not been established.

Anti-inflammatory analgesics used in rheumatic disorders

Phenylbutazone (*Butazolidin*)
Dose 400–600 mg orally, daily, preferably after meals—reduce after a few days to half this dose. Suppositories 250 mg at night.
   An effective analgesic and anti-inflammatory agent used in rheumatoid arthritis, gout, ankylosing spondylitis and other musculoskeletal disorders. Its severe side effects mean, however, that it must be used with great caution and for short periods only.

Adverse effects. Phenylbutazone may cause gastric irritation and gastro-intestinal bleeding. It causes sodium, chloride and fluid retention. The increase in plasma volume can cause cardiac failure and pulmonary oedema. Skin rashes can also occur and fatal blood dyscrasias have also been reported. *Contraindications.* Phenylbutazone should be avoided in patients with oedema, hypertension and hepatic disease. It interacts with warfarin, other anti-coagulants and anti-diabetic drugs such as tolbutamide and chlorpropamide.

Oxyphenbutazone (*Tanderil*)
Similar in action and adverse effects to phenylbutazone.

Indomethacin (*Indocid*)
This has analgesic anti-inflammatory and antipyretic properties similar in effect to phenylbutazone. Used in musculoskeletal disorders, such as ankylosing spondylitis, osteoarthritis, rheumatoid arthritis and acute gout.

Adverse effects. Headache, giddiness, faintness, nausea and vomiting. Patients who operate or drive machinery must be careful when taking indomethacin. It may cause gastric ulceration and bleeding. Psychiatric disturbance such as confusion, depression and depersonalization also occur. Prolonged use can result in eye damage. *Contraindications*: peptic ulcer, renal and hepatic disease, psychiatric disorders and the elderly.

Other anti-inflammatory analgesic preparations
Azapropazone (*Rheumox*), Diclofenac (*Voltarol*), Diflunisal (*Dolobid*), Fenbufen (*Lederfen*), Fenclofenac (*Flenac*), Fenoprofen (*Fenopron*), Feprazone (*Methrazone*), Flurbiprofen (*Froben*), Ibuprofen (*Brufen*), Ketoprofen (*Orudis*), Naproxen (*Naprosyn, Synflex*), Piroxicam (*Feldene*), Sulindac (*Clinoril*).

Other drugs used in rheumatic disorders

In rheumatoid arthritis, not responsive to anti-inflammatory analgesics, other drugs may be used which are not analgesics, but have a specific anti-rheumatoid effect. Corticosteroids (Chapter 13), immunosuppressants (Chapter 18), and chloroquine (Chapter 23) are all drugs that are sometimes used.

Gold (sodium aurothiomalate) (*Myocrisin*)
Dose weekly intramuscular injections up to 50 mg.
   Action uncertain, but no benefit is apparent until at least two months therapy has been given.

Adverse effects. Skin reactions and blood dyscrasias. Urine should be tested regularly for proteinuria.

Penicillamine (*Cuprimine, Distamine*)
Dose increase gradually to 250 mg–1 g orally daily.
   Similar delayed response as for gold. Also used in cystinuria and Wilson's disease (where it acts by removing excess copper).

Adverse effects. Hypersensitivity, skin reactions, blood dyscrasias. Urine should be tested regularly for proteinuria.

Drugs used in the treatment of gout

Gout is a painful inflammatory condition characterized by elevated plasma uric acid levels and deposits of uric acid crystals in the joints. In an acute attack of gout, anti-inflammatory drugs such as indomethacin and phenylbutazone may be used.

Colchicine
Dose 1 mg initially, followed by 500 micrograms every two to three hours until pain is relieved.

Although not an analgesic, colchicine is effective in the treatment of acute gout.

Adverse effects. Gastrointestinal upset, renal damage and blood dyscrasias.

Probenecid (*Benemid*)
Dose 500 mg–2 g in divided doses.

Probenecid is used in the prophylaxis of gout since it increases the excretion of uric acid by the kidney. A high fluid intake is essential with this drug in order to avoid crystallization in the urine. Often given in conjunction with colchicine.

Adverse effects. Has few adverse effects, but nausea and vomiting may occur.
Ethebenecid (*Urelim*) and Sulphinpyrazone (*Anturan*) are other uricosuric drugs.

Allopurinol (*Zyloric*)
Dose 200–400 mg orally in divided doses.

Acts by blocking uric acid synthesis. Often used in conjunction with colchicine and uricosuric drugs.

Adverse effects. Rashes, hypersensitivity reactions, including fever.

NARCOTIC ANALGESICS

Opium
Opium is obtained from the unripe capsule of the poppy, *Papaver somniferum*. Nowadays purified alkaloids are extracted for medicinal use.

Pharmacology
Enkephalins are physiological neurotransmitters which act

on specific receptors in the brain, spinal cord and gut. Opiates are effective by acting on these receptors, which inhibit the transmission of pain and certain other impulses. The main pharmacological effects are:

(a) *Pain* is relieved by an action on the receptors in the brain and spinal cord. Opiates are the most powerful analgesics.
(b) *Euphoria* is produced by an action on brain receptors.
(c) *Respiration.* Opiates decrease the sensitivity of the respiratory centre in the brain stem to carbon dioxide, causing depression of respiration, and possibly apnoea, especially in patients with respiratory failure. The cough reflex is also depressed.
(d) *Hypotension* may occur owing to depression of the vasomotor centre in the brain stem.
(e) *Constipation* is produced by an action on gut opiate receptors, which increase the tone and decrease the motility of smooth muscle.
(f) *Nausea and vomiting* by a central action.
(g) *Constriction* of the pupil.
(h) *Tolerance* develops after regular use. If opiates are withdrawn the endogenous enkephalins are then ineffective and the withdrawal syndrome develops consisting of anxiety, muscle twitching, sweating, diarrhoea, hyperventilation and tachycardia.
(i) *Addiction* is due to mental dependence on the euphoriant effects of morphine, and fear of withdrawal syndrome.

Therapeutic uses. The main use of opiates is to relieve severe pain in conditions of limited duration, e.g. postoperatively or myocardial infarction and in conditions where addiction is of no concern, e.g. terminal illness.

Other uses include cough suppression, the treatment of diarrhoea and symptomatic relief in left ventricular failure.

There are no clear categories under which to describe the

narcotic compounds. Here they are rather arbitrarily grouped according to their general effects.

Morphine group

Morphine is a powerful analgesic and euphoriant, but has great potential for addiction. It is well-absorbed but is extensively metabolized. It can be given intramuscularly or even intravenously for a rapid effect. It is used as an analgesic: in association with anaesthesia, following injury or operation, in medical conditions such as myocardial infarction, and in the terminal stages of diseases such as cancer. In the former instances, addiction is unlikely as the drug is used for a limited time, and in the latter ceases to be of importance. Small doses of morphine are effective in obstetrics and post-operative pain relief, given epidurally, probably by acting on receptors in the spinal cord and avoiding many of the side effects of morphine.

Small doses of morphine are used in cough sedatives and anti-diarrhoeal preparations.

Adverse effects. Dependency and respiratory depression are the major side effects. Nausea and vomiting are frequent, and constipation may be troublesome with chronic use, as in terminal illness. Overdosage may be recognized by drowsiness leading rapidly to unconsciousness, pinpoint pupils, cyanosis and apnoea. Death may be prevented by intravenous naloxone (an opiate antagonist).

Contraindications. Morphine is contraindicated in patients with marked liver disease, myxoedema or respiratory disease.

If used in patients with head injuries it will affect the pupil reactions which are used to monitor the patient. Patients receiving monoamine oxidase inhibitors should not be given morphine, since hypertension, excitation and occasionally coma may be produced.

Morphine passes the placental barrier and may predispose to fetal asphyxia if given too near the time of delivery.

Morphine
Dose 10–40 mg orally, 5–15 mg subcutaneously or intramuscularly.

Diamorphine hydrochloride (Heroin)
Dose 10–40 mg orally, 5–10 mg intramuscularly or intravenously.

Papaveretum (*Omnopon*)
Dose 10–20 mg parenterally.

Kaolin and morphine mixture
Dose 10 mg orally.
   A mixture given to control diarrhoea.

Codeine group
Codeine is the next most important alkaloid of opium, having about one-sixth of the analgesic potency of morphine.
   It is used as a cough suppressant and anti-diarrhoeal agent. Dihydrocodeine is used as an analgesic.

Codeine phosphate
Dose 10–60 mg.
   An anti-diarrhoea preparation.

Codeine linctus
Dose 5 ml. (15 mg codeine phosphate).
   A cough sedative.

Dihydrocodeine tartrate (*DF 118*)
Dose 30–60 mg orally or intramuscularly.

Methadone

Methadone, a synthetic analgesic, is used in controlling morphine withdrawal symptoms since it is metabolized very slowly and avoids abrupt opiate withdrawal. Also used in the management of severe pain in terminal illness.

Contraindications. As for morphine.

Methadone Hydrochloride (*Physeptone*)
Dose 5–10 mg orally or subcutaneously.

Pethidine

Pethidine is a synthetic substance related chemically to atropine, but has similar properties to morphine. It is used in obstetrics and in the treatment of renal and biliary colic and post-operatively. Side effects are similar to those of morphine.

Pethidine hydrochloride
Dose 25–100 mg (tablets or injection)

Other opiates

Ethoheptazine
Dose 75–150 mg orally.

Dextromoramide (*Palfium*)
Dose 5–20 mg orally or parenterally.
  An analgesic similar to morphine and pethidine.

Pentazocine (*Fortral*)
Dose 30–60 mg injection (or 25–100 mg orally).

Buprenorphine (*Temgesic*)
Dose 300–500 micrograms by injection or sublingually.

Dextropropoxyphene (*Distalgesic*)
32.5 mg and paracetamol 325 mg. A popular analgesic for
minor conditions but may be rapidly fatal in overdosage due
to dextropropoxyphene-induced respiratory depression.

Dipipanone (*Diconal*)

Phenoperidine (*Operidine*)

Opiate antagonists

These block the opiate receptors and completely reverse the
effects of opiates. The older antagonists, such as nalorphine,
have some opiate-like activity, and have been superseded by
naloxone, which is a pure antagonist. Naloxone is used in
opiate overdosage, but since the effect is shorter than most
opiates, repeated injections may be required.

Naloxone (*Narcan*)
Dose 0.4–1.2 mg intravenously.

HYPNOTICS

A hypnotic is a drug given to induce sleep. A sedative will
induce drowsiness and a tranquillizer will produce calmness.
In practice, however, the differences in effect are often dose-
related and many drugs can serve all three purposes.

   The routine administration of hypnotics to patients in
hospitals is to be deprecated. In patients with insomnia, a
reason should be sought and often simple nursing measures
will achieve the desired result. The problems associated with
hypnotics include:

1. Suppression of normal REM or paradoxical sleep which
    is marked by an increase in rapid eye movements,
    respiration and body movements. REM sleep occurs for
    about 20 min in every hour and seems essential for a

restful night's sleep. If the hypnotic is suddenly withdrawn a 'rebound' phenomenon can occur, where the person experiences disturbed sleep and nightmares for some weeks. Hypnotics, therefore, should always be withdrawn slowly.

2. A 'hangover' effect is commonly experienced the following day, and some impairment of performance should also be expected.
3. They tend to cause confusion in the elderly and should be avoided.
4. The problem of dependency means that they should be used for short periods only.
5. They potentiate the effects of alcohol, which should be avoided.

Barbiturates

Barbiturates are salts and derivatives of barbituric acid. Their action can be understood by examining the successive stages of their depressant effect on the central nervous system.

At sub-hypnotic doses they are sedatives. At three to five times the sedative dose they will produce sleep, while in larger doses they will produce anaesthesia and coma. A further increase in dosage can produce depression of the respiratory and vasomotor centres in the medulla, resulting in death.

As with all hypnotics, tolerance can develop, while psychic and physical dependence can occur with prolonged use. Sudden withdrawal of barbiturates can produce agitation, tremor, restlessness and convulsions. Withdrawal must be phased over several weeks and with a gradual reduction in dosage. The long-acting barbiturates, such as phenobarbitone, can cause accumulative toxicity with drowsiness, slurred speech, 'drunken' like behaviour and sedation. Skin bullae and rashes are sometimes seen at toxic levels. They also cause enzyme induction in the liver, so that drugs such as anticoagulants and phenytoin are metabolized much more quickly. Drugs such as alcohol and tranquillizers can potentiate the action of barbiturates. Used as a hypnotic they cause the 'rebound' phenomena, confusion in the elderly and a 'hangover' effect the following morning.

The problems resulting from the use of barbiturates as sedatives and hypnotics would seem to outweigh their value. The introduction of the benzodiazepines and other tranquillizers indicate little justification for the continuing use of barbiturates. They still retain a place as short-acting anaesthetics and as potent anticonvulsants.

The length of action of the barbiturates is dependent upon the rate at which they are metabolized in the liver.

Phenobarbitone
This has a long half life of several days, so it tends to have a cumulative action. It is now rarely used as a hypnotic, but remains an effective anticonvulsant.

Intermediate and short-acting barbiturates
Although shorter-acting than phenobarbitone, they still tend to have a cumulative action. Their effects last two to six hours. Their use as hypnotics is now no longer recommended.

Preparations include amylobarbitone sodium (*Sodium Amytal*), butobarbitone (*Sonergan, Soneryl*), pentobarbitone (*Nembutal*), cyclobarbitone (*Phanodorm*), cyclobarbitone calcium (*Rapidal*), hexobarbitone (*Evipan*), quinalbarbitone (*Seconal*), quinalbarbitone sodium 50 mg with amylobarbitone sodium 50 mg (*Tuinal*), heptabarbitone (*Medomin*).

Ultra-short-acting-barbiturates
The ultra-short-acting barbiturates produce unconsciousness within seconds if injected intravenously. They are a very effective means of inducing anaesthesia in minor surgical procedures and prior to electroconvulsive therapy.

Thiopentone sodium (*Pentothal, Intraval*)
This causes a smooth 'induction' and rapid anaesthesia, but it also causes necrosis of subcutaneous tissue and thrombus formation if injected into an artery.

The use of barbiturates as anaesthetics is discussed in Chapter 10.

Other hypnotics

Chloral hydrate
Dose Hypnotic 500 mg–1.6 g orally
       Sedative 250 mg–1 g three times a day
Chloral hydrate is a sedative and hypnotic which is readily dissolved in water. Derived from ethyl alcohol, it is one of the oldest known hypnotics. It induces sleep in 15–30 min and maintains its effect for six–eight hours, producing little 'hangover' effect.

It is particularly useful with children and the elderly and is available as a paediatric chloral elixir.

Adverse effects. Chloral hydrate is a gastric irritant and may produce allergic reactions. It has an additive effect with alcohol.

Triclofos sodium
Dose 1–2 g.
Similar to chloral hydrate, but with less gastric irritation.

Dichloralphenazone (*Welldorm*)
Dose 650–1300 mg.
A preparation of chloral and phenazone given in tablet form. It has less gastric irritant effect than chloral hydrate.

Paraldehyde
Dose 5–10 ml. orally or intramuscularly. Can also be given rectally in normal saline.

The action of paraldehyde on the central nervous system is similar to that of chloral. It is an oily liquid with a characteristic and unpleasant odour. It is a powerful hypnotic which is excreted in the urine and by the lungs. It reacts with plastics and should be given in a glass syringe. Its tendency to cause abscess formation when injected intramuscularly means that the same site should not be used twice. Paraldehyde is used in status epilepticus, severe agitation, and alcohol withdrawal states.

Chlormethiazole (*Heminevrin*)
Dose 500 mg–1 g orally as hypnotic
      500 mg three times daily as sedative
      250 mg intravenous infusion followed by 8 mg/min, depending on patient response.
Related to thiamine, it is effective in preventing alcohol and drug withdrawal symptoms. Can produce sedation in confused and agitated patients, particularly the elderly. It can, however, produce dependence, so is not recommended for routine use, as a sedative or hypnotic.

Can be given intravenously in status epilepticus but thrombophlebitis may occur.

Adverse effects. Conjunctivitis and sneezing can occur and in high doses may cause respiratory depression. *Contra-indications:* barbiturates and alcohol potentiate the effects of chlormethiazole with resulting respiratory and cardiovascular depression.

Methyprylone (*Noludar*)
Dose 200–400 mg orally.

Glutethimide (*Doriden*)
Dose 500 mg orally.

Nitrazepam (*Mogadon*)
Dose 5–10 mg at night.
   One of the benzodiazepines used more often as a hypnotic rather than anxiolytic. It may produce a 'hangover' effect next day. Nitrazepam has a long half life, so accumulation may occur. As with other hypnotics, it may produce rebound phenomena and tolerance can develop.

Flurazepam (*Dalmane*)
Dose 30 mg at night.

Temazepam (*Normison*)
Dose 10–30 mg.
   A benzodiazepine, with a shorter half life, so accumulation effects are less, with little 'hangover' effect or drowsiness the following day.

Triazolam (*Halcion*)
Dose 125–250 micrograms.
   Has a very short half life, with similar advantages to those of temazepam.

ANTICONVULSANTS

These drugs are used in the treatment of epilepsy, which is due to the spread of abnormal electrical discharge across the brain. Epileptic fits due to hypoglycaemia, hypocalcaemia or fevers may cease with treatment of the causative conditions. In most cases, however, the only treatment is prophylactic by administration of anticonvulsant drugs. They do not in themselves cure epilepsy. Treatment is usually long-term, but the drug may be gradually withdrawn after three years without a fit, although convulsions may recur.

Pharmacology. The action of anticonvulsant drugs is unknown. One view speculates that anticonvulsants suppress activity in neurones adjacent to an epileptogenic focus, thus blocking the spread of the electrical discharge. Another view is that anticonvulsant drugs raise the threshold of excitability of all neurones, that is, they can tolerate greater excitation without a fit being precipitated.

Therapeutic uses. Effectiveness in controlling fits is closely related to the plasma concentration of anticonvulsants. Below an optimal plasma level, the effectiveness of the drug is less. Above this level the severity of side effects increases without greater control of fits being achieved. Therefore, monitoring plasma concentrations is useful to maintain the correct dosage.

It is now realized that the majority of convulsions can be controlled as adequately with a single drug, as with multiple drug therapy, and the likelihood of drug interactions is thus diminished.

Anticonvulsant therapy can be divided into three categories:

1. Treatment of generalized and focal seizures (which involve loss of consciousness with generalized convulsions).
2. Treatment of absences (with no loss of consciousness) in children.
3. Treatment of status epilepticus (series of seizures without the regaining of consciousness between each fit).

Treatment of generalized seizures

Phenytoin sodium (*Epanutin, Dilantin*)
Dose 100–400 mg orally in a single daily dose. Therapeutic plasma level 10–20 micrograms/ml.

Phenytoin is probably the drug of choice for the treatment of generalized seizures. Unlike phenobarbitone, it has very little hypnotic action and does not cause general depression of the central nervous system.

Adverse effects. Phenytoin may produce gastro-intestinal disturbances, ataxia, nystagmus, skin rashes, gum hypertrophy, hirsutism, acne, and, less commonly, peripheral neuropathy. Phenytoin causes folic acid deficiency, resulting in megaloblastic anaemia, which may be rectified by regular administration of folic acid. Phenytoin also interferes with vitamin D metabolism and thus occasionally causes osteomalacia. Phenytoin is a potent inducer of hepatic enzymes and decreases the effect of oral anticoagulants.

Phenobarbitone
Dose 100–300 mg in a single evening dose. Therapeutic plasma level 10–30 micrograms/ml.

Phenobarbitone is the longest-acting barbiturate, its effects lasting for several days after cessation of treatment. It is only slowly absorbed.

Adverse effects. Skin rashes, ataxia or drowsiness may occur in some individuals, while in others restlessness and agitation may prevail. It is a more powerful enzyme-inducer than phenytoin, and decreases the effect of oral anticoagulants.

Primidone (*Mysoline*)
Dose 500–1500 mg orally daily in divided doses.

Primidone is metabolized to phenobarbitone, and probably has little independent anticonvulsant activity. Therefore, it may have no advantage over phenobarbitone.

Adverse effects. As for phenobarbitone.

Carbamazepine (*Tegretol*)
Dose 400–1600 mg orally daily in divided doses. Therapeutic plasma level 4–10 micrograms/ml.

Probably the drug of choice in psychomotor and focal epilepsy. Also used in trigeminal neuralgia.

Adverse effects. Gastro-intestinal disturbances, ataxia, drowsiness, skin rashes, and rarely, jaundice, leucopenia and aplastic anaemia. Carbamazepine is a potent inducer of enzymes.

Clonazepam (*Rivotril*)
Dose 1–8 mg orally in a single evening dose.
   Very similar to other benzodiazepines, such as diazepam. Mostly used for the treatment of childhood myoclonic seizures and infantile spasms. Drowsiness is common with higher doses, and limits its usefulness.

Preparations used in the treatment of absences

Sodium valproate (*Epilim*)
Dose 800 mg–2.5 g orally daily. Therapeutic plasma level 60–100 micrograms/ml. However, its effectiveness may bear little relation to the plasma concentration.
   It is the drug of choice for absences, but also very effective in generalized seizures.

Adverse effects. Gastro-intestinal disturbances, occasionally sedation, weight gain and alteration in hair texture. Rarely, fatal hepatic necrosis has occurred with high doses.

Ethosuximide (*Zarontin*)
Dose 500–2000 mg daily.

Adverse effects. Mild gastro-intestinal disturbance.

Troxidone (*Tridione*)
Dose 1–2 g daily in divided doses.
   Now only a third-choice drug for absences.

Preparations used in the treatment of status epilepticus

Diazepam (*Valium*)
Dose 10 mg intravenously or rectally as necessary.

The effects of the first few boluses may only last 20 min, owing to distribution, but eventually a prolonged effect, for several days, may be obtained, owing to the slow elimination of diazepam.

Clonazepam, chlormethiazole, paraldehyde and even thio-pentone have also been useful.

Treatment of status epilepticus may cause sufficient respiratory depression to necessitate artificial ventilation.

DRUGS USED IN PARKINSON'S DISEASE

Parkinsonism is a condition characterized by rigidity, tremor and hypokinesia. It is caused by an imbalance of the neutrotransmitters dopamine and acetylcholine in the corpus striatum and basal ganglia of the brain. In this condition acetylcholine with its excitatory function predominates over the inhibitor dopamine.

Drug treatment is aimed at redressing this imbalance either by increasing the level of dopamine (dopaminergic) or alternatively reducing acetylcholine (anticholinergic). In the case of drug-induced Parkinsonism, symptoms disappear when the drug is stopped. Drug treatment does not affect the progression of the disorder, but merely alleviates some of the symptoms.

Dopaminergic drugs

Levodopa
Dose 125 mg twice-daily increasing to a maximum of 8 g daily.

This drug, a precursor of dopamine, is converted to dopamine in the brain.

Therapeutic use. In most patients improvement in rigidity and hypokinesia takes several months to appear, though tremors are relatively unaffected.

Adverse effects. Nausea and vomiting (lessens when administered with food), orthostatic hypotension, involuntary movements and psychiatric disturbances, such as restlessness, hallucinations, delusions and sleep disturbances may occur.

Levodopa and carbidopa (*Sinemet*)
Carbidopa inhibits the conversion of levodopa to dopamine outside the brain, thus reducing some of the side effects such as nausea, vomiting and postural hypotension.

Levodopa and benserazide (*Madopar*)
Similar to levodopa and carbidopa.

Bromocriptine (*Parlodel*)
Similar to, but more expensive than, levodopa.

Amantadine (*Symmetrel*)
Dose initially 100 mg daily increasing to maximum of 400 mg daily.
    Compared with levodopa, its effect is rapid, but unpredictable.

Adverse effects. These include psychiatric disturbances, such as insomnia, irritability, dizziness, hallucinations and epilepsy. Other side effects include oedema and livedo reticularis.

Anticholinergic drugs
These drugs block the effects of acetylcholine.

Therapeutic uses. They may lessen rigidity and reduce tremors, though have little effect on hypokinesia. These drugs may be used in drug-induced Parkinsonism.

Adverse effects. Psychiatric disturbances may occur, such as confusion and hallucinations. Other side effects include constipation, dry mouth, difficulty in focussing and difficulty in micturation.

Benzhexol (*Artane*)
Dose 2–5 mg orally three times daily.

Benztropine (*Cogentin*)
Dose 1–2 mg orally at bedtime.
   This drug may cause drowsiness.

Procyclidine (*Kemadrin*)
Dose 2.5–20 mg orally daily.

Orphenadrine (*Disipal*)
Dose 200–400 mg daily.
   This drug may cause a degree of euphoria.

DRUGS USED FOR SPASTICITY

These drugs are used to reduce muscle spasticity that occurs following injury to or disease of the spinal cord. They are much less useful in spasticity due to cerebral damage. Since they act at different sites, combined drug therapy may be beneficial.

Diazepam (*Valium*)
Dose 2–60 mg daily orally.
   Acts on the central nervous system. Higher doses produce drowsiness, but tolerance to this may occur. Other benzo-diazepines (Chapter 11) may also be effective.

Baclofen (*Lioresal*)
Dose 15–100 mg daily orally in divided doses.
Inhibits spinal-cord reflexes. Dose should be increased gradually.

Adverse effects. Vomiting, drowsiness, delirium, epilepsy, hypotension.

Dantrolene (*Dantrium*)
Dose 25 mg daily, increasing over several weeks up to 300 mg daily in divided doses.
Acts directly on skeletal muscle. It takes several weeks to produce the maximal effect.

Adverse effects. Dizziness, weakness, diarrhoea, rashes and hepatic dysfunction.

AMPHETAMINES

The drugs of the amphetamine group stimulate the cortex causing increased level of arousal. They stimulate the respiratory centre and suppress the appetite.

Therapeutic uses. Amphetamines are rarely used in medicine. However, they may be used to treat narcolepsy and are sometimes used to treat hyperkinesis where they calm the child and decrease hyperactive behaviour. Amphetamine and amphetamine-like drugs have a limited use in weight reduction in combination with other measures, such as diet and group support.

Adverse effects. Agitation (though in the case of fenfluramine, sedation), insomnia and restlessness are likely to occur. Another side effect is gastro-intestinal disturbances. Users are liable to develop dependency.

Amphetamine sulphate (*Benzedrine*)
Dose 5–20 mg orally.

Dexamphetamine sulphate (*Dexedrine*)
Dose 5–20 mg.

Phentermine (*Duromine*)
Dose 15–30 mg in the morning.
   Used as an appetite suppressant.

Diethylpropion (*Apisate, Tenuate*)
Dose 75 mg.
   Used as an appetite suppressant.

Fenfluramine (*Ponderax*)
Dose 1–2 capsules daily.
   Used in obesity. Abrupt withdrawal may induce depression.
Dependance is less likely than with the other drugs.

9 Drugs Affecting the Autonomic Nervous System

Drugs which act on the autonomic nervous system do so by either 'mimicking' (agonists) or inhibiting (antagonists) the effects of acetylcholine or noradrenaline, the principle neurotransmitters involved in the system.

PARASYMPATHETIC (CHOLINERGIC) DRUGS

Acetylcholine

This is released from the synaptic terminals in preganglionic fibres of both the sympathetic and parasympathetic systems, and in postganglionic parasympathetic fibres.

Nicotinic actions

(a) Stimulation of parasympathetic ganglia
(b) Stimulation of sympathetic ganglia
(c) Contraction of skeletal muscle

Note that (b) is mediated via the sympathetic system, and (c) by the peripheral nerves.

Muscarinic actions

(a) Secretory (e.g. sweat, intestinal, pancreas, etc.)
(b) Smooth-muscle contraction (bronchi, gut, bladder)
(c) Sphincter relaxation (gut, bladder, also evacuation)

(*d*) Miosis (pupils constrict)
(*e*) Bradycardia

Acetylcholine agonists

Carbachol
Dose 0.25 mg subcutaneously, 1.4 mg orally.
  Carbachol is a synthetic compound resembling acetylcholine but has a longer duration of action. It stimulates the bladder and bowel and is used post-operatively and after childbirth. It may cause hypotension and diarrhoea.

Bethanechol (*Myotonine*)
Dose 10–30 mg orally three to four times daily. 2.5–5 mg by subcutaneous injection.
  Bethanechol is similar to carbachol.

Pilocarpine
Pilocarpine is used to constrict the pupils in glaucoma.

ANTICHOLINESTERASES

These are drugs which inhibit the action of cholinesterase, an enzyme responsible for the breakdown of acetylcholine. They therefore potentiate the effects of acetylcholine. Their use is largely confined to the treatment of myasthenia gravis, an autoimmune disease causing muscle weakness and fatigue by reducing acetylcholine release where motor nerves stimulate skeletal muscle (called the motor endplate).

Neostigmine (*Prostigmin*)
Dose 75–300 mg orally daily. 1.2–5 mg by subcutaneous, intramuscular or intravenous injection.
  Neostigmine is used in the diagnosis (a single test dose will produce rapid, if transient, improvement) and treatment of

myasthenia gravis. Also useful in relieving paralytic ileus and severe constipation and for its myotic effect on the eye. Also used by anaesthetists to reverse the effects of muscle relaxants (Chapter 10).

Adverse effects. These are mainly muscarinic in effect and include nausea, excessive salivation, sweating, intestinal colic, diarrhoea and bradycardia. Atropine may help prevent these effects. Excessive dosage will produce muscle weakness, similar to myasthenia, due to constant stimulation of the muscle.

Physostigmine (*Eserine*)

Physostigmine is effective in the treatment of glaucoma but has been replaced by neostigmine in the treatment of myasthenia gravis.

Edrophonium chloride (*Tensilon*)

Dose 5–10 mg intravenously as test dose.

This preparation is related to neostigmine. When injected intravenously, it will produce a temporary improvement in muscle weakness. It is used as a diagnostic test for myasthenia gravis.

Pyridostigmine bromide (*Mestinon*)

Dose 5–25 mg orally three to four times daily.

Pyridostigmine is similar to neostigmine but is longer-acting.

Ambenonium chloride (*Mytelase*)

Dose 5–25 mg three to four times daily.

Distigmine bromide (*Ubretid*)

Dose 5–20 mg daily orally.

Acetylcholine antagonists

These can be divided into three main groups according to their actions.

1. Anticholinergics
2. Ganglion blockers
3. Neuromuscular blocking agents

1. Anticholinergics

Anticholinergic drugs block the muscarinic effects of acetylcholine at postganglionic receptor sites.

Atropine

Dose 600 micrograms–1.2 mg orally or by injection.

Atropine is derived from the *Atropa Belladonna* (Deadly Nightshade) plant or is manufactured synthetically.

Effects. (*a*) Reduces bronchial, gastric and salivary secretions, causing a dry mouth. (*b*) Reduces vagal tone to the heart, causing an increase in heart rate. These effects make it useful as a pre-anaesthetic agent. (*c*) Relaxes smooth muscle in the gut, bladder and bronchi. It has been used in the past as a bronchodilator and to relieve colonic spasm and to treat peptic ulcers. (*d*) Mydriatic and cycloplegic (paralyses ciliary muscles of the eye (see Chapter 21).

Atropine also has an initial stimulating, then depressant, effect on the central nervous system. This is only obvious in overdose, when insomnia, restlessness and hallucinations may occur.

Adverse effects. These are essentially those related to its antimuscarinic effects, e.g. dry mouth, tachycardia, flushing, difficulty in micturition, constipation and occasionally contact dermatitis.

Homatropine
Homatropine is used solely as a mydriatic (see Chapter 21).

Hyoscine (Scopolamine**)**
Dose 300–600 micrograms four times daily orally or by subcutaneous injection.

Hyoscine exerts the same antimuscarinic effects of atropine, but also has a strong central nervous system depressant action, inducing sedation and sleep. It has been used to treat peptic ulceration, spastic colon, and to relieve muscle rigidity in Parkinson's disease. It also has an anti-emetic effect, making it useful in treating nausea and vertigo, and especially travel-sickness. Hyoscine can be used on its own as pre-medication, or combined with morphine or pethidine. It has similar adverse effects to atropine.

Hyoscine butylbromide (*Buscopan***)**
Dose 20 mg orally four times daily or 20 mg by intramuscular or intravenous injection.

Buscopan has been used in the treatment of colonic spasm and dysmenorrhoea.

Dicyclomine hydrochloride (*Merbentyl, Ovol, Debendox***)**
Dose 30–60 mg orally in divided doses.

Dicyclomine is a useful anti-emetic.

The value of other anticholinergics used as antispasmodics is discussed in Chapter 4.

2. Ganglion blockers
Drugs in this group block acetylcholine at both sympathetic and parasympathetic ganglia. The main effect is to lower blood pressure. They are considered in Chapter 5.

3. Neuromuscular blocking agents
By blocking or interfering with the effects of acetylcholine at

the neuromuscular junction in skeletal muscle, these drugs cause a muscular paralysis. They include suxamethonium, tubocurarine and gallamine and are considered in Chapter 10.

SYMPATHETIC (ADRENERGIC)

Noradrenaline is the main neurotransmitter released from the postganglionic synaptic terminals of the sympathetic nervous system. The varied effects of noradrenaline can be understood by considering the different postsynaptic receptor sites to which it binds. These are alpha (α) and beta (β_1 and β_2) receptors. Note that noradrenaline and adrenaline are also released from the adrenal medulla.

1. Alpha adrenergic effects
(*a*) Arteriolar constriction
(*b*) Mydriasis

Agonists
Noradrenaline and adrenaline.

Antagonists
Phenoxybenzamine, phentolamine and tolazoline.

Note that there is also a group of drugs classified as postganglionic blockers, which prevent the *release* of noradrenaline from sympathetic postganglionic nerve endings. These are bethanidine, guanethidine, debrisoquine and guanoclor, and are discussed in Chapter 5.

2. Beta-1—adrenergic effects
(*a*) Tachycardia
(*b*) Increased myocardial contractility
(*c*) Increased myocardial irritability

Agonists
Noradrenaline, adrenaline, isoprenaline, dopamine and dobutamine.

Antagonists
Practolol, propranolol, oxprenolol, acebutolol, atenolol and metoprolol.

3. Beta-2—adrenergic effects
(*a*) Smooth-muscle relaxation (bronchi, gut, uterus, muscle, arteries)
(*b*) Sphincter constriction

Agonists
Adrenaline, isoprenaline and salbutamol.

Antagonists
Propranolol and labetalol.

4. Metabolic effects
Glycogenolysis and lipolysis.

All these drugs are discussed fully in Chapters 5 and 6.

DRUGS USED IN THE TREATMENT OF MIGRAINE

Treatment of the acute attack

Ergotamine tartrate (*Cafergot, Femergin, Lingraine*)
Dose 1–2 mg orally or sublingually. Also available as an inhaler and suppositories.

Ergotamine will cause contraction of all smooth muscle in the bronchi, intestine and uterus. Although an adrenergic antagonist, it will also produce vasoconstrictions in arterioles. This effect on the cranial arteries will relieve the headache of migraine. Repeated administrations may cause gangrene, withdrawal headaches and angina. Other side effects include nausea, vomiting and abdominal pain. Its use in obstetrics is described in Chapter 19.

Contraindications. Pregnancy, hypertension, peripheral arterial disease, angina.

Dihydroergotamine (*Dihydergot*)
Dose 2–3 mg orally repeated every 30 min if required. 1–2 mg by intramuscular or subcutaneous injection.
This preparation is less effective than ergotamine but has fewer side effects.

Isometheptene mucate
Dose 1–2 capsules up to six times daily.
Midrid contains isometheptene (similar in action to adrenaline), dichloralphenazone and paracetamol.

Other drugs
Symptomatic relief is provided, as appropriate, by analgesics (Chapter 8), e.g. aspirin; anti-emetics (Chapter 4), e.g. metoclopramide; or tranquillizers (Chapter 11), e.g. diazepam.

Drugs used in the prophylaxis of migraine

Clonidine (*Dixarit*)
Dose 50–100 micrograms orally daily.
Normally used in the treatment of hypertension, it reduces the responsiveness of cranial arteries.

Pizotifen (*Sanomigran*)
Dose 500 micrograms–3 mg orally daily.
Pizotifen is a serotonin antagonist.

Methysergide (*Deseril*)
Dose 1–2 mg orally daily.

Methysergide is also antiserotonergic in action but its value is limited in migraine, because of its severe side effects. These include drowsiness, nausea, oedema and, most importantly, retroperitoneal fibrosis.

Beta-blockers
Drugs such as propranolol and acebutolol are also effective in preventing migraine attacks in some patients.

10 Anaesthetics and their Adjuncts

Anaesthesia is associated with, in varying degrees, narcosis, muscle relaxation and analgesia. To achieve this a combination of drugs is usually given rather than one single substance.

ADJUNCTS TO ANAESTHESIA

Premedication

Prior to anaesthesia, certain drugs are given to lessen anxiety, to facilitate easier induction and maintenance of anaesthesia, and to inhibit the production of mucous stimulated by inhaled anaesthetics. Opiates may be given to allay fear, while atropine diminishes bronchial secretion. Phenothiazines potentiate sedatives as well as acting as an anti-emetic, and are commonly used. Narcotics are also used to increase analgesia during anaesthesia.

Neuromuscular blocking agents

These drugs produce muscle relaxation which could only otherwise be achieved from very much larger doses of anaesthetics. Since all skeletal muscles are affected, including the intercostals and the diaphragm, artificial respiration is a necessary consequence. They act by blocking the receptors on skeletal muscle, opposite the nerve endings, thus preventing acetylcholine causing muscular contraction. These effects can be antagonized by increasing acetylcholine concentrations, by inhibiting cholinesterase (which is responsible for its breakdown) with cholinesterase inhibitors (e.g. neostigmine)

(Chapter 9). The dose of neostigmine (*Prostigmin*) is 2.5–5 mg intravenously, preceded by atropine 1 mg intravenously to prevent acetylcholine causing dangerous bradycardia. Malignant hyperthermia is a rare, but serious, adverse effect.

Tubocurarine (*Tubarine, Jexin***)**
Dose 5–15 mg intravenously.
 This drug is a purified alkaloid of curare; it produces paralysis of the voluntary muscles in about four minutes and remains active from half to one hour. It causes a rash due to the release of histamine, and transiently blocks the autonomic ganglia, causing a lowering of blood pressure.

Gallamine triethiodide (*Flaxedil***)**
Dose 80 mg intravenously.
 It acts in 1½ min and the effect lasts 15–25 min.

Pancuronium bromide (*Pavulon***)**
Dose initially 50–100 micrograms/kg intravenously.
 Quicker onset of action than tuborcurarine, with no histamine-releasing or autonomic-blocking actions. Widely used for major surgery, and for ventilated patients in intensive care units.

Alcuronium chloride (*Alloferin***)**

Fazadinium bromide (*Fazadon***)**

Suxamethonium bromide (*Scoline, Brevidil***)**
Dose 40–100 mg intravenously.
 Paralysis lasts only five minutes. It differs from other neuromuscular blocking drugs by first causing muscle contraction and it therefore cannot be reversed by anti-cholinesterases, and paralysis is preceded by muscle twitching, which may cause muscle pains. It is destroyed by cholin-

esterase, and deficiency of this enzyme may result in prolonged paralysis.

Other adjuncts

The use of narcotics for their analgesic effect has already been mentioned (also Chapter 8). After anaesthesia, their effects may require reversal with naloxone (*Narcan*) (Chapter 8), or doxapram (*Dopram*) may be used to reverse respiratory depression only (Chapter 6). Sometimes, bleeding during operation is reduced by lowering the blood pressure with hypotensive drugs (Chapter 5).

GENERAL ANAESTHETICS

Intravenous anaesthetics

Thiopentone (*Pentothal***)**
Dose may vary between 100–500 mg given intravenously in a 2.5% solution or as a 10% solution per rectum.

Thiopentone is presented as a yellowish powder which is mixed with sterile water prior to use. It is a quick-acting barbiturate producing a pleasant loss of consciousness. It is seldom given as a sole anaesthetic as it provides little analgesia. Therefore, it is usually given with other drugs, thereby providing additional analgesia as well as maintaining anaesthesia. Thiopentone is considered well 'tried and trusted' and has been in use for over 30 years.

Therapeutic uses. Used to produce anaesthesia for short procedures such as electroconvulsive therapy, to produce a light narcosis for local analgesia, and to induce anaesthesia, maintained by other agents. Given intravenously, it acts within half a minute and the anaesthesia lasts for three to four minutes. Thiopentone may also be given rectally in the treatment of status epilepticus. Artificial ventilation is always necessary owing to respiratory depression.

Adverse effects. Injection into tissue may result in necrosis and ulceration of the subcutaneous tissue. Injection into an artery will result in thrombosis and eventually gangrene. Cardiovascular depression and laryngeal spasm may occur. Since the plasma half life is about 48 hours, patients should avoid driving and taking other drugs, including alcohol, which may cause sedation, for up to 24 hours following anaesthesia.

Methohexitone sodium (*Brietal*)
Dose 1 mg/kg intravenously in a 1% solution.

This drug is a similar barbiturate to thiopentone, though shorter-acting and three times more potent. The main difference is that the plasma half life is between one and two hours compared with thiopentone's 48 hours. The patient's rapid recovery makes it suitable for use in outpatient departments.

Propanidid (*Epontol*)
Dose 5–10 mg/kg in 5% solution.

Propanidid is an ultra-short-acting anaesthetic. Onset of anaesthesia may be accompanied by hyperventilation followed by hypoventilation and occasionally apnoea lasting up to half a minute. It is preferred to barbiturates for outpatient procedures, since patients may go home sooner.

Adverse effects. Hypersensitivity common, especially broncho-spasm.

Alphaxolone and alphadolone (*Althesin*)
Dose 0.05–0.1 ml./kg intravenously.

This mixture of two steroids results in anaesthesia in one

'arm–brain' circulation time and recovery (which is pleasant) 5–10 min later. It is used for short surgical procedures or as a general induction agent.

Adverse effects. Hypersensitivity and bronchospasm common.

Ketamine (*Ketalar*)
Dose 8–10 mg/kg intramuscularly, 2 mg/kg intravenously.

When injected intravenously, anaesthesia is established within thirty seconds and lasts 5–8 min. Given intramuscularly, loss of consciousness occurs after 3 min and recovery after 30 min. Transition to full consciousness is rapid, and though often accompanied by unpleasant dreams (especially in adults) these may be lessened by allowing a longer period of quietness or by administering diazepam.

Ketamine produces loss of consciousness with analgesia without producing muscle relaxation. The advantage of this is that the patient's airway can be easily maintained. Respiration and blood pressure are not depressed by ketamine. The drug is useful for procedures such as short operations, cardiac catheterization and dressing of burns in children, but is less useful in adults.

Diazepam (*Diazemuls, Valium*)
Dose 5–50 mg intravenously.

Can be used as an alternative to thiopentone, and causes less respiratory depression, but recovery is usually longer. Widely used for minor procedures such as electrical cardioversion and gastroscopy. Lorazepam (*Ativan*) is an alternative benzodiazepine.

Inhalational anaesthetics
The depth of unconsciousness produced is related to the partial pressure of the anaesthetic carried in the blood. As the

diffusion of the anaesthetic gas is not resisted by the alveoli in the lungs, its partial pressure is determined largely by the solubility of the anaesthetic in the blood. Where there is low solubility, only a small amount of gas is absorbed resulting in a rapid rise in alveolar concentration and blood partial pressure. These gases cause rapid anaesthesia in the patient and also effect a rapid recovery. The converse is true of the relatively highly soluble drugs which have a slower rise in alveolar concentration and blood partial pressure.

Recovery is also dependent on an effective blood supply removing the drug from the central nervous system. It is eliminated from the blood via the lungs and kidneys or metabolized in the liver or stored temporarily in fatty tissues.

Nitrous oxide (N_2O)

Stored in a blue cylinder (in UK) under 50 atmospheres at 28°C. Previously known as 'laughing gas'.

A good analgesic, though to be effective as an anaesthetic it needs to be combined with an anaesthetic drug. Inhalation is often preceded by intravenous induction of anaesthesia and it is usually administered with oxygen in the ratio 7:3. Nitrous oxide may also be combined with a volatile agent such as halothane.

Therapeutic uses. Apart from its use with other anaesthetics during surgery, it is also used in conditions that require analgesia such as labour, following myocardial infarction, and for burn dressings. These other procedures are carried out without loss of consciousness, using nitrous oxide and oxygen alone, in the ratio 1:1 (*Entonox*), which can be self-administered.

Adverse effects. Struggling and excitement may occur on induction. Prolonged administration (over 48 hours) may produce bone marrow depression.

Cyclopropane
Stored in an orange cylinder (in UK) under 75 lb/in^2 at 28°C.

It is a very potent anaesthetic requiring only a small amount, which allows a high percentage of oxygen to be administered with it. As it is relatively insoluble in blood, induction of and recovery from anaesthesia is rapid. Cyclopropane is usually administered via a closed circuit because of its explosive nature and expense.

Therapeutic use. Used particularly in patients with heart disease where oxygenation is poor.

Adverse effects. Cyclopropane causes depression of the respiratory system, usually requiring assisted ventilation, and may precipitate dysrhythmias.

Cyclopropane has been largely replaced by halothane.

Diethyl ether
Stored in sealed dark bottles in a cool place.

This anaesthetic is a colourless and very volatile liquid with an unpleasant odour. It is highly inflammable and decomposes on exposure to air, light and heat. Stabilizing substances, e.g. hydroquinone, are added to inhibit decomposition. Diethyl ether is preferably administered via a closed circuit, particularly where electrical equipment is present.

After initial stimulation, diethyl ether depresses the central system. However, it has a high safety margin. As diethyl ether is a soluble compound it produces slow induction of, and recovery from, anaesthesia, and an inducing drug should be used.

Therapeutic use. Although now rarely used in modern operating theatres, it is still useful where facilities are limited, owing to its ease of administration and safety margin. In these circumstances, ethyl chloride may be used as an inducing drug, and ether administered as drops onto gauze held over the mouth and nose.

Adverse effects. Diethyl ether may cause hyperglycaemia and convulsions in febrile patients. It is irritant to the respiratory tract, and there is a high incidence of vomiting.

Halothane (*Fluothane*)

Halothane is currently the most commonly used volatile anaesthetic drug. It is a colourless liquid with a musty smell. It is non-explosive, non-inflammable and non-irritant. Halothane decomposes on exposure to light, though it remains stable when combined with soda-lime. Its low solubility results in rapid induction of, and recovery from, anaesthetic.

It is usually administered with an oxygen–nitrous-oxide mixture in a semi-open circuit, though it can be given in a closed circuit.

Therapeutic use. Used particularly in major surgery.

Adverse effects. Higher doses necessitate assisted ventilation, and may induce arrhythmias, bradycardia and vasodilatation. It can cause hepatitis, especially after repeated administration.

Methoxyflurane (*Penthrane*)

Methoxyflurane is a colourless liquid, non-explosive and non-inflammable with a characteristic fruity odour. Induction of, and recovery from, anaesthesia is slow due to its high solubility and the difficulty in vapourizing. Respiratory depression may necessitate assisted ventilation.

Adverse effect. Higher doses induce renal toxicity.

Trichlorethylene (*Trilene*)

Though naturally colourless, a blue dye is added for identification purposes. It is non-inflammable, non-explosive and has a sweetish smell. It decomposes on exposure to heat and light and in contact with soda-lime. Therefore it cannot be used in a closed circuit. Since the blood solubility is high, induction of, and recovery from, anaesthesia are slow.

Therapeutic uses. Commonly used with nitrous oxide and oxygen during surgery. Trichorethylene has good analgesic properties and may be used to relieve pain in labour, and during painful procedures.

Adverse effects. Post-operative nausea, vomiting and headache.

Enflurane (*Ethrane***)**
Similar to, but quicker-acting than, halothane, and causes fewer cardiac arrhythmias.

LOCAL ANAESTHETICS

Local anaesthetics block the impulse passing along the sensory and motor nerve fibres. However, pain fibres are more easily blocked, and touch and movement may be spared. Depending on the site of injection, they may either block the nerve supply to the area or may affect the nerve endings. It may also be administered by being sprayed or painted onto mucous membranes, instilled into the eye, or given epidurally.

The effectiveness of local anaesthetic drugs lasts from five minutes to two hours, and the time may be prolonged by the addition of adrenaline 1–200 000 (which causes capillary constriction and so prevents rapid removal of the anaesthetic).

Adverse effects. Stimulation of the central nervous system may occur if there is excessive blood concentration, resulting in anxiety, tremor and possibly convulsions. Direct injection into a blood vessel may cause circulatory collapse.

Cocaine
Dose 5% for cornea, 10% for nose and throat.

This drug is an alkaloid of coca leaves and is a powerful local anaesthetic readily absorbed by mucous membrane and raw surfaces.

Therapeutic uses. It is of value when used in the eye as it blanches the sclera, dilates the pupil and anaesthetizes superficial eye structures. It facilitates the removal of foreign bodies from the eye, after which the eye must be covered. It is also used on the mucous membranes of the nose and throat.

Adverse effects. Cocaine can produce circulatory collapse in sensitive individuals even when applied locally, and a test dose should first be given. Absorption occurs readily, and excessive doses may cause confusion, arrhythmias, vomiting, convulsions and formication (a sensation of crawling on the skin). It is a drug of addiction.

Lignocaine (*Xylocaine, Lidothesin*)
Dose 0.5–2% for infiltration.

The most commonly used local anaesthetic. Its effect lasts for 15–45 min. Lignocaine injection is available with adrenalin, and as a solution, gel, jelly, ointment, cream, lozenges, and spray for topical application.

Procaine
Similar to, but shorter-acting, and less effective than lignocaine.

Amethocaine
It is effective when applied to mucous membrane or instilled into the eye, but lignocaine may be a safer alternative.

Benzocaine
A weak local anaesthetic, used topically to relieve irritation and pain in the mouth and anus.

Cinchocaine (*Nupercaine, Dermacaine*)
Available as a cream or ointment for minor skin conditions.

Mepivacaine (*Chlorocain*)
Used in epidural and spinal anaesthesia. It has a slightly longer action than lignocaine.

Prilocaine (*Citanest*)
Similar to lignocaine. It can be used in regional intravenous analgesia after restricting the blood flow temporarily to the forearm with a cuff (Bier's block). Higher doses may cause methaemoglobinaemia.

Bupivacaine (*Marcain*)
This drug is a long-acting potent local anaesthetic. As an epidural analgesic in labour, its effects last 2–4 hours (dose up to 150 mg four-hourly).

11 Drugs used in Mental Illness

In the absence of any understanding of specific biochemical abnormalities in psychiatric illness, all psychopharmacological methods of treatment are empirical. Psychotrophic drugs, i.e. drugs that affect thought, mood or behaviour, are rarely curative on their own and will deal with only a part of the patient's total psychological disturbance.

Most of the range of psychotrophic drugs now available have been developed in the past 30 years. Previous to this it was only possible to treat anxious, psychotic or other disturbed patients by giving drugs (e.g. barbiturates, paraldehyde) which produced a sedative or hypnotic effect. Now modern tranquillizers will produce calmness, and reduce aggression and tension, without inducing sleep. Neuroleptic drugs (those used in the treatment of severe mental disturbance or psychoses) may also have a more specific antipsychotic action by controlling delusions, hallucinations, thought disturbance and motor overactivity without clouding consciousness. This allows the patient to be more amenable to other forms of non-pharmacological therapy.

Inappropriate prescribing of psychotrophic drugs can often cause iatrogenic disorders in themselves. Nurses must therefore carefully monitor patients receiving these drugs and be specially alert to the occurance of adverse effects.

MAJOR TRANQUILLIZERS

These are alternatively described as neuroleptic or antipsychotic drugs.

Pharmacology. They block receptors in the central nervous system, preventing the rapid dispersal of neurotransmitters. Psychoses are associated with the presence of low concentrations and an imbalance of neurotransmitters in the brain. Major tranquillizers block brain dopamine and other neurotransmitter receptors, which may contribute to their therapeutic effect and explain some of their adverse effects.

Therapeutic uses. Major tranquillizers are used mainly in the treatment of psychosis and have a calming effect with a comparatively low level of sedation. They are also used in the short term in acute confusional states.

Adverse effects. They enhance the effect of analgesics, hypnotics and alcohol. Jaundice may result from blocking of bile canaliculi in the liver. Parkinsonian features are common owing to dopamine blocking action on the basal ganglia, and oro-facial writhing movements may occur after long-term therapy. Anticholinergic drugs used for Parkinson's disease (Chapter 8) are often given to counteract Parkinsonian features. Postural hypotension can occur owing to blockage of alpha-adrenergic receptors. Impairment of temperature regulation may cause hypothermia—especially in the elderly. Hypersensitivity skin reactions and blood dyscrasias may occur.

Nurses administering chlorpromazine may develop contact dermatitis, and so should wear gloves and avoid spray from the needle.

Phenothiazine group
This group of tranquillizers is commonly used in the treatment of psychotic states. Some of the drugs within this group are used for their anti-emetic properties and others for their antipruritic qualities.

Chlorpromazine (*Largactil, Chloractil, Dozine***)**
Dose 75–300 mg daily. May be given orally, intravenously

or intramuscularly.

It is introduced gradually, increasing to a maintenance dose of 75–300 mg daily. However, much larger doses—up to 1000 mg daily—may be given to psychotic patients.

Therapeutic uses. In psychiatry it is used to treat psychomotor over-activity in manic organic states and schizophrenia. In general medicine, it is used for the relief of restlessness and agitation.

Promazine (*Sparine*)
Dose 50–800 mg orally.

Less potent than chlorpromazine, and only used for minor psychoses.

Promethazine (*Phenergan*)
Dose 25–75 mg orally.

Used as a premedication, as an anti-emetic and anti-histamine.

Thioridazine (*Melleril*)
Dose 30–600 mg orally in divided doses.

Popular for the elderly for confusional states.

Trifluoperazine (*Stelazine*)
Dose 2–150 mg orally intramuscularly.

Used for acute and chronic psychotic states, and as an anti-emetic.

Fluphenazine enanthate (*Moditen*)
Used for psychoses, especially schizophrenia, and available as a depot preparation requiring intramuscular injections as infrequently as monthly (*Modecate, Moditen Enanthate*). An initial test dose should first be given.

Perphenazine (*Fentazin*)

Prochlorperazine maleate (*Stemetil, Vertigon*)
Used as an anti-emetic.

Pericyazine (*Neulactil*)

Thiopropazate (*Dartalan*)

Thioproperazine (*Majeptil*)

Diphenyldibutylpiperidine group

Pimozide (*Orap*)
Dose 2–10 mg once daily.
   A popular drug for schizophrenia, similar to chlorpromazine, but less sedative.

Fluspirilene (*Redeptin*)
Dose 2–20 mg intramuscularly weekly.
   For schizophrenia.

Thioxanthines group

Flupenthixol (*Depixol*)
Dose 20–40 mg every two to four weeks intramuscularly.
Initial test dose of 20 mg, then 20–40 mg after five–ten days.
   An antipsychotic drug, which, like pimozide, has a mood-elevating effect which is useful for psychotic withdrawn patients, e.g. for chronic schizophrenia.

Chlorprothixene (*Taractan*)
Dose 30–400 mg daily orally.

Clopenthixol (*Clopixol*)
Dose 100–400 mg intramuscularly every two to four weeks, after a test dose.
  Used for chronic schizophrenia, especially agitated patients.

Thiothixene

Oxpertine (*Integrin*)
Dose 40–120 mg three times daily as an antipsychotic, 10 mg three times daily for anxiety states.
  Structurally different from the thioxanthines.

Butyrophenones

Haloperidol (*Serenace, Haldol*)
Dose 0.5–10 mg three times daily.
  Used in the management of manic and schizophrenic states.

Droperidol (*Droleptan*)
Dose 5–20 mg orally, intravenously or intramuscularly.

Benperidol (*Anquil*)

Trifluperidol (*Triperidol*)

MINOR TRANQUILLIZERS

Benzodiazepine group

Pharmacology. They affect the limbic system, acting on specific receptors. Most benzodiazepines have a half life of two days; therefore a single daily dose is usually adequate at night-time.

Therapeutic uses. These drugs are used mainly in the treatment of anxiety states. They are also used as hypnotics, sedatives or anticonvulsants. Inappropriate use for depression or personality disorders will be detrimental to the patient.

Adverse effects. Given orally, side effects are uncommon, although ataxia and dizziness may occur, particularly in the elderly. They also potentiate the effect of drugs which affect the central nervous system, e.g. alcohol. For these reasons it is advised that patients on minor tranquillizers avoid the use of alcohol and handling machinery or driving. Overdosage rarely causes serious respiratory depression, in contrast to barbiturates.

Chlordiazepoxide (*Librium*)
Dose 10–100 mg orally.
   Tranquillizing effect on patients with anxiety, tension or fear without a marked sedative effect.

Diazepam (*Valium, Atensine*)
Dose 5–30 mg orally.
   Diazepam has a similar action to chlordiazepoxide, though it has a wider range of application. It is particularly useful in the treatment of status epilepticus (5–10 mg intravenously) (Chapter 8) and is used as an intravenous anaesthetic (Chapter 10).

Oxazepam (*Serenid-D*)
Dose 15 mg three times daily, orally.

Medazepam (*Nobrium*)
Dose 15–30 mg daily, orally.

Lorazepam (*Ativan*)
Dose 2–10 mg daily, orally for anxiety states, 2–4 mg

parenterally as premedication or an anaesthetic.
    Has a shorter half life than most benzodiazepines.

Clorazepate (*Tranxene*)
Dose 15 mg daily, orally.

Clobazam (*Frisium*)
Dose 20–60 mg orally daily.

Hydroxyzine (*Atarax*)
Dose 75–400 mg daily, orally.

Meprobamate (*Equanil, Miltown*)
Dose 1.2–2.4 g daily.
    Not a benzodiazepine. Can cause serious respiratory
depression in overdosage.

ANTIDEPRESSANT DRUGS

Mood is related to the concentration of amines (noradrenaline,
5-hydroxytryptamine, etc.) in the brain, and a depressed
mood occurs secondary to a reduction in these amine levels.
Antidepressant drugs increase brain amine levels, and can
elevate a depressed mood with a corresponding improvement
in associated depressive symptoms.
    Antidepressants are classified by their mode of action into
two main groups:

1. Monoamine oxidase inhibitors (MAOI)
2. Tricyclic compounds, and related drugs

    In general, they have a slow onset of action and prolonged
effect. Elimination from the body is by metabolism in the
liver.

Monoamine oxidase inhibitors (MAOI)

Monoamine oxidase (MAO) is an enzyme responsible for the breakdown of adrenaline, noradrenaline and other amines in nerve endings. MAOI irreversibly block this enzyme and cause accumulation of amines, both within and outside the central nervous system.

Therapeutic uses. MAOI are now only used in the few patients with severe depression unresponsive to other drugs and electroconvulsive therapy. Their onset of action is slow (about 14 days). Concurrent administration of L-tryptophan (a precursor of 5-hydroxytryptamine) may increase their effectiveness.

Phenelzine (*Nardil*)
Dose 30–60 mg daily.

Isocarboxazid (*Marplan*)
Dose 20–40 mg daily.

Tranylcypromine (*Parnate*)
Dose 20–40 mg daily.

Iproniazid (*Marsilid*)
Dose 25–50 mg daily.

Adverse effects. MAOI increase noradrenaline levels in the sympathetic nervous system and cause constipation, dry mouth, blurred vision and difficulties with ejaculation and micturition. Postural hypotension causing dizziness and fainting is common. Rashes, insomnia, agitation, convulsions and liver damage can occur.

Drug interactions. MAOI potentiate the actions of tricyclic antidepressants, pethidine, barbiturates, antihistamines, alcohol, antiparkinsonian drugs, insulin, tolbutamide, and hypotensive drugs like guanethidine. Hypertension and excitation can occur with methyldopa.

Potentially the most catastrophic interaction occurs with drugs such as amphetamines, proprietary cold cures, slimming aids and foods (such as cheese, broad beans, red wine, Marmite) which contain tyramine or dopamine. These substances release the adrenaline and noradrenaline which accumulates in patients taking MAOI, resulting in a sudden hypertensive crisis with pounding headache, vomiting and occasionally cerebral haemorrhage. Patients taking MAOI should carry a card describing their treatment, and should be given a list of drugs and foods to avoid.

Contraindications. MAOI should not be used in patients with liver disease, cerebrovascular disorders or epilepsy. Their use in other patients is restricted by the potential severity of drug interactions or side effects.

Tricyclic and related compounds

These drugs are effective antidepressants, and are also used in obsessional and phobic states. Although used in childhood enuresis, there is a risk of serious poisoning should the child take an accidental overdosage. Imipramine (*Tofranil*) was the prototype of these antidepressants. It increases the level of noradrenaline and 5-hydroxytryptamine by blocking re-uptake into the presynaptic nerve. There is a two to three week delay before the drug takes effect. The dose ranges from 10 mg to 150 mg daily, the elderly usually requiring lower doses. Since the plasma level can vary enormously in different individuals on identical doses, blood-level monitoring may be helpful if available. Because of the long half life a once-daily night-time dose is adequate for treatment. To prevent relapse after the depressive illness, prolonged maintenance treatment may be of benefit.

Adverse effects, As with the MAOI, atropine-like anticholinergic effects are common and include dry mouth,
constipation, blurred vision and urinary retention; hypotension, especially in the elderly, tremor, nausea and vomiting
can also occur. Some tolerance occurs to the anticholinergic
effects. Cardiac arrhythmias may occur in patients with heart
disease, and convulsions in patients predisposed to epilepsy.
Overdosage causes respiratory depression, convulsions and
cardiac arrhythmias.

Drug interactions. The tricyclics are incompatible with
MAOI and a three-week period should elapse between
discontinuing a patient on MAOI and commencing tricyclics.
They are antagonistic to the hypotensive action of guanethidine,
bethadine and clonidine, and have an additive sedative effect
with alcohol and other sedatives.

Contraindications. They should be avoided if possible in
patients with heart disease, epilepsy, glaucoma or prostatism.

Desipramine (*Pertofran***)**
Dose 75–200 mg daily.

Trimipramine (*Surmontil***)**
Dose 50–100 mg daily.

Clomipramine (*Anafranil***)**
Dose 50–150 mg daily. Can also be given by intravenous
infusion.

Amitriptyline (*Tryptizol, Lentizol***)**
Dose 75–200 mg daily.

Nortripyline (*Aventyl***)**
Dose 75–200 mg daily.

Doxepin (*Sinequan*)
Dose 75–100 mg daily.

Butriptyline (*Evadyne*)
Dose 75–150 mg daily.

Dibenzepin (*Noveril*)
Dose 320–400 mg daily.

Dothiepin (*Prothiaden*)
Dose 75–150 mg daily.

Iprindole (*Prondol*)
Dose 90–180 mg daily.

Protriptyline (*Concordin*)
Dose 15–60 mg daily.

Tetracyclic and other antidepressants
These are new compounds with similar action to that of the tricyclics. They have fewer cardiac and anticholinergic side effects. Viloxazine and nomifensine may also have anti-convulsant properties.

Maprotiline (*Ludiomil*)
Dose 50–150 mg daily.

Mianserin (*Bolvidon, Norval*)
Dose 30–60 mg daily.

Viloxazine (*Vivalan*)
Dose 100–300 mg daily.

Nomifensine (*Merital*)
Dose 50–150 mg daily.

Trazodone (*Molipaxin*)
Dose 100–600 mg daily.

L-tryptophan (*Optimax, Pacitron*)
Dose 3–6 g daily.
   An amino-acid, which may be of some value in depression. Causes drowsiness. May be given with other antidepressants or MAOI.

Lithium carbonate
(*Camcolit, Priadel, Liskonum*)
Lithium is an alkali metal similar to sodium and potassium. It exerts a mood stabilizing effect and can be used in the treatment of acute mania, although its lengthy delay in acting (one to two weeks) will usually require that a tranquillizing drug also be used. Its main value lies in the prophylaxis of bipolar (manic depressive) and unipolar (recurrent depressive) illness.

Pharmacology. Since toxicity occurs at a plasma concentration little higher than that required for therapy, a careful check should be kept on the plasma concentration. Lithium should always be started at a low dosage until a therapeutic level is reached, usually a plasma concentration of 0.5–1.5 mmol/litre. Above 2 mmol/litre toxic effects may appear. Normally 750–2000 mg per day will be required in divided doses, or once-daily if given in the slow-release form.
   A life-long maintenance dose may be required in patients with recurrent manic depression.

Adverse effects. Early and common side effects include nausea, diarrhoea and fine tremor which often disappear after two to six weeks. At therapeutic plasma levels, polyuria, polydipsia and weight gain can occur but may improve with a slight reduction in dosage. Plasma levels above the therapeutic range can produce hypothyroidism, drowsiness, coarse tremor, ataxia, vomiting, diarrhoea and dysarthria. The drug should be stopped immediately, otherwise coma and death may ensue.

Drug interactions. Thiazide diuretics can cause lithium retention and toxicity. It can be administered safely with tricyclic and related compounds, but should be given with caution in patients receiving neuroleptic drugs.

Contraindications. Lithium should not be administered to patients with a history of serious renal or cardiac disease or hypothyroidism. It is advisable to assess renal and thyroid function before commencing lithium treatment.

12 Histamine and Antihistamines

HISTAMINE

Histamine is released from cells in many allergic conditions. Acting on H_1 receptors, it increases bronchial secretions, dilates capillaries and increases their permeability (causing swelling), dilates cerebral vessels (causing headache), causes a fall in blood pressure, and contraction of bronchial smooth muscle (precipitating asthma). These last two effects are prominent and may rapidly cause death in anaphylactic shock, when allergic reactions release large amounts of histamine. However, other factors, such as the slow-reacting substance of anaphylaxis (SRS-A) and kinins are probably more important in precipitating asthma and anaphylaxis; hence the ineffectiveness of antihistamines in these conditions.

Acting on H_2 receptors, histamine causes secretion of gastric acid and pepsin.

Histamine has no diagnostic or therapeutic uses.

ANTIHISTAMINES

H_1 antagonists

These drugs are commonly referred to as 'antihistamines'. They are most effective when used prior to histamine release (i.e. prophylactically). They also have therapeutic activity unrelated to histamine antagonism. They are well absorbed when given orally, and are metabolized by the liver. Most of them are effective for 12–24 hours after a single dose.

Therapeutic uses

1. As histamine antagonists, they suppress the symptoms of certain allergic conditions such as hay fever, acute urticaria and angioneurotic oedema. They are useless in asthma, anaphylaxis and chronic urticaria.
2. Most antihistamines are potent anti-emetics and are useful against motion sickness, radiation sickness and drug-induced vomiting. They can also be used against nausea and vomiting in pregnancy, but only those compounds, such as dicyclomine, which, by long usage, are known to be safe in this situation, should be used.
3. Most antihistamines cause drowsiness and can be used for sedation, e.g. pre-operatively.

Preparations available

	Dose per day (mg)
Mepyramine (*Anthisan*)	50–100
Chlorpheniramine (*Piriton*)	4–16
Diphenhydramine (*Benadryl*)	25–75
Cyclizine (*Marzine*)	50–150
Promethazine (*Phenergan*)	25–50

Many other preparations are available, but none has any particular advantages. Although the daily dosage is usually divided into three or four doses, a single daily dose is often effective. This is best given in the evening, since all antihistamines cause drowsiness. Parenteral and topical preparations are available, but the latter are ineffective, may cause skin reactions, and should not be used.

Adverse effects. Drowsiness is very common; patients should be advised not to drive or operate machinery and should avoid other sedatives such as alcohol or hypnotics. Dizziness, diplopia, gastrointestinal upsets and tinnitus may occur. Many antihistamines produce anticholinergic side effects (Chapter 9). They can cause convulsions in epileptics, or if taken in overdosage. Their actions are prolonged and exaggerated in severe liver disease, and should be avoided.

H_2 antagonists

Cimetidine (*Tagamet*) is commonly used—ranitidine (*Zantac*) is a recent alternative. They prevent the formation of gastric acid and are used in the treatment of chronic peptic ulcer. Oral cimetidine (400 mg twice a day) suppresses ulcer symptoms, and promotes healing, usually within two months. A reduced dose (400 mg at night) is often given for a further year to prevent relapse. Intravenous cimetidine has been tried in acute gastro-intestinal haemorrhage, but only seems to be effective in special circumstances.

Adverse effects. Generally mild, and include diarrhoea, myalgia, skin rashes and dizziness. Confusion and gynae-comastia occur rarely, especially in the elderly and patients with renal failure, for whom the dosage should be reduced.

14 Hormones and Allied Substances

Hormones are the secretions of the endocrine glands which occur naturally in the body and are responsible for controlling body functions. Many different hormones are given in the treatment of disease, often as replacement for natural secretions, where there is under-production from a gland. Included in this chapter are synthetic alternatives for replacement therapy, and drugs which inhibit the production of hormones where there is over-secretion.

THYROID

Thyroxine sodium (*Eltroxin***)**
Dose 50–300 micrograms daily orally.

Used in replacement therapy for thyroid deficiency, i.e. hypothyroidism (cretinism and myxoedema). The dosage should be increased only every two weeks, especially in the elderly and patients with heart disease. The effects of the drug last for over one week.

Liothyronine sodium (*Tertroxin***)**
Dose 10–100 micrograms daily orally or intravenously.

More rapidly metabolized, but quicker acting than thyroxine. Thyroxine is preferable for maintenance treatment.

Antithyroid drugs
These are effective in hyperthyroidism (thyrotoxicosis), by

blocking the incorporation of iodine into thyroxine, in the thyroid gland. They are usually effective within two weeks, but a high dosage must be given initially in divided doses. Beta-adrenergic blockers, such as propranolol, are sometimes also given initially to help control symptoms. After six weeks, when the patient is euthyroid, the dosage may be gradually reduced, and need only be given once daily. To reduce the chance of relapse, treatment should be continued for 18 months, unless radio-iodine treatment or surgery are contemplated. Antithyroid drugs may unpredictably precipitate agranulocytosis, which is usually reversible; therefore patients should be told to report immediately any fever or sore throat. A goitre may increase in size during the initial stages of treatment.

Carbimazole (*Neo-Mercazole*)
Dose initially 30–60 mg, reducing to 5–20 mg daily.
Usually the first-choice antithyroid drug. May also cause skin rashes.

Propylthiouracil
Dose initially 200–600 mg, reducing to 50–200 mg daily.
An alternative to carbimazole, if that drug produced skin rashes.

Potassium perchlorate (*Peroidin*)
Dose initially 600 mg–1 g daily, reducing to 300–500 mg daily.
Now only used if other antithyroid drugs are not tolerated. May cause aplastic anaemia. Acts by preventing iodine uptake.

Aqueous iodine solution
Dose 0.5 ml. three times daily; contains 5% iodine and 10% potassium iodide.

Often given for two weeks prior to thyroidectomy, as an alternative to antithyroid drugs. If given to patients treated with potassium perchlorate, may precipitate thyrotoxicosis.

PARATHYROID

Calcitonin
Dose 50–100 units daily intramuscularly or intravenously.

Blood calcium is increased by parathyroid hormone, and lowered by calcitonin. The latter is used to lower blood calcium concentrations in some patients with dangerous hypercalcaemia (especially due to malignant disease), and to treat severe Paget's disease. Salmon calcitonin (*Calsynar*) is less immunogenic than porcine calcitonin (*Calcitare*) and is preferred for long-term treatment.

Calcium gluconate
Dose 10 ml. of a 10% solution slowly intravenously.

Several oral preparations of calcium salts are available, and although they may occasionally be of value in hypoparathyroidism, their usefulness is unclear. Severe hypocalcaemia can be corrected with intravenous calcium gluconate, but the effect is short-lived. Hypoparathyroidism is usually treated with vitamin D preparations alone.

ADRENOCORTICAL HORMONES

The cortext of the adrenal gland produces a number of hormones with similar chemical structure, called steroids. They predominantly have effects on metabolism and immune responsiveness (glucocorticoids) and sodium and water retention by the kidney (mineralocorticoids). Some steroids affecting sexual characteristics are also produced. Hydrocortisone (cortisol) is the principal natural glucocorticoid, and aldosterone the major natural mineralocorticoid, although hydrocortisone also has considerable mineralocorticoid activity.

Mineralocorticoid effects

There is retention of sodium and water, associated with an increased excretion of potassium, causing hypokalaemia.

Therapeutic uses. As replacement therapy in Addison's disease. In this condition, there is adrenal cortical destruction, and consequently renal loss of sodium and water, causing hypotension. This is reversed by mineralocorticoids. Hydrocortisone, given as glucocorticoid replacement, has a significant salt-retaining effect, but a small dose of a more powerful mineralocorticoid is required in addition.

Deoxycortone pivalate (*Percorten*)

Dose 50–100 mg every two to four weeks by intramuscular injection.

A depot mineralocorticoid for use in Addison's disease.

Fludrocortisone (*Florinef*)

Dose 50–200 micrograms orally daily.

Given as replacement therapy together with glucocorticoids, in Addison's disease.

Glucocorticoid effects

Excessive endogenous hydrocortisone production occurs in Cushing's syndrome. There is decreased glucose utilization by the tissues, causing insulin resistance, hyperglycaemia and glycosuria. There is protein catabolism, causing muscle wasting, osteoporosis, growth retardation in children, skin atrophy and bruising. There is increased fat on the face, shoulders and abdomen. The inflammatory response and allergic reactions are suppressed, masking the signs of

infection. Psychoses may occur with high doses. The mineralocorticoid actions of excessive hydrocortisone cause oedema
and hypertension.

Withdrawal symptoms. Normally, hydrocortisone secretion
by the adrenals is controlled by adrenocorticotrophic hormone
(ACTH), which is secreted by the pituitary. Prolonged
treatment with corticosteroids, especially high doses, suppresses ACTH secretion. Consequently, if steroid treatment
is suddenly stopped, or there is an intercurrent illness
requiring increased endogenous hydrocortisone secretion,
there will be adrenocortical insufficiency. This may result in
vomiting, unconsciousness, cardiovascular collapse and arthralgia. Therefore, severe illness, accident or operation in a
patient taking steroids, or within a year of stopping a
prolonged course, may necessitate supplementary hydrocortisone. All patients being treated with steroids should
carry a card with the steroid dosage on, and should warn their
doctors of this.

Symptoms may also occur on stopping steroids, owing to
recrudescence of the disease being treated. The problems of
steroid withdrawal may be ameliorated by reducing the
steroid dosage gradually.

Therapeutic uses. Hydrocortisone and cortisone are used as
replacement therapy in Addison's disease. Otherwise, steroids
are used to suppress many diseases, by their anti-inflammatory
effect. These include asthma, sarcoidosis and allergic alveolitis;
collagen diseases, especially systemic lupus erythematosus;
ulcerative colitis, Crohn's disease and chronic active hepatitis;
hypersensitivity reactions; the nephrotic syndrome; uveitis
and iritis; cerebral oedema; many skin diseases; haematological
conditions, such as auto-immune haemolytic anaemia, idio-
pathic thrombocytopaenia, lymphoid leukaemia and lymph-
oma.

Adverse effects. These are common, dose-related, and may be severe. They are a consequence of drug-induced Cushing's syndrome and steroid-withdrawal, both of which have just been discussed. Dyspepsia is also common.

Systemic, but not local, side effects may be reduced by topical application, such as: enemas for ulcerative colitis; inhalation for asthma; eye drops for iritis; local applications for skin diseases; injections into joints in rheumatoid arthritis.

Cortisone acetate (*Cortelan, Cortistab, Cortisyl*)
Dose for replacement therapy 25–37 mg orally daily.

Hydrocortisone (*Hydrocortistab, Hydrocortone*)
Dose for replacement therapy 20–30 mg orally daily.

This is the most important glucocorticoid secreted naturally and is preferred for replacement therapy. With serious intercurrent illness or surgical operations in patients with hypoadrenalism, higher doses of the sodium phosphate (*Efcortesol*) or succinate salts (*Efcortelan, Solu-Cortef*) (100–500 mg intramuscularly or intravenously six-hourly) may be required. These doses of parenteral hydrocortisone are also used to treat severe steroid-responsive diseases, such as severe asthma. Hydrocortisone is also available as ointments, creams, eye-drops, lozenges, suppositories and enemas, for topical application, and as hydrocortisone acetate injection for joints and tendons.

Prednisolone (*Codelcortone, Deltacortril, Precortisyl, Prednisol, Sintisone*)
Dose up to 100 mg daily, for anti-inflammatory effect, for which it is five times more potent that hydrocortisone.

Except for replacement therapy, and intravenous therapy, it is preferred to hydrocortisone, since it causes much less salt and water retention.

Prednisone (*Decortisyl, Deltacortone***)**
Dose up to 100 mg daily.

   It is converted to prednisolone in the body, and has similar indications.

Methylprednisolone (*Medrone***)**
Similar to prednisolone, but often used intravenously, or as a long-acting intramuscular preparation (*Depo-Medrone*).

Triamcinolone (*Adcortyl, Kenalog, Ledercort, Lederspan***)**
More potent anti-inflammatory effect than prednisolone, but may cause particularly severe muscle wasting.

Dexamethasone (*Decadron, Dexacortisyl, Oradexon***)**
Dose up to 16 mg daily.

   More potent than prednisolone, causing even less salt and water retention.

Betamethasone (*Betnelan, Betnesol***)**
Similar to dexamethasone.

Cortisone synthesis inhibitor

Metyrapone (*Metopirone***)**
Dose 750 mg four-hourly orally for six doses.

   Metyrapone is used to assess pituitary and adrenal functions, by inhibiting cortisol production in the adrenal. The reduced blood cortisol concentrations result in increased ACTH production by the anterior pituitary, if it is functioning satisfactorily, and plasma ACTH can be measured. ACTH in turn stimulates the adrenal gland to produce excess 17-oxogenic steroids, which are prevented from becoming cortisol by the metyrapone. These steroids can be measured in the urine.

ADRENAL MEDULLA

The medulla produces mainly adrenaline. Noradrenaline is also produced by the medulla, and, more importantly, by sympathetic nerves, and increases blood pressure, by constricting arterioles, and increases the heart rate. Adrenaline is released in response to stress, and increases the heart rate, raises the blood pressure, increases blood sugar and dilates bronchioles. Despite this, no illness results from absent adrenal medullary secretion.

Adrenaline

Dose 0.2–0.5 ml. subcutaneously or intramuscularly for acute anaphylaxis. It may be given intravenously, only for asystolic cardiac arrest. Since cardiac arrhythmias are common, there are no other indications for parenteral adrenaline. Also used topically to prevent bleeding from the nose, mouth and throat, and as eye-drops.

PANCREAS
Insulin

Insulin is produced by the beta-cells of the Islets of Langerhans. This hormone controls the blood sugar by increasing the uptake of glucose by muscle and liver, and its incorporation into starch. It also increases proteins and fat synthesis.

Failure of the pancreatic beta-cells results in diabetes mellitus, with hyperglycaemia. The main use of insulin is in the treatment of diabetes mellitus, but it is also used to produce hypoglycaemia, as a test, usually of pituitary function. Since insulin is destroyed by gastric secretions, it must be injected.

Although it can be made synthetically, commercially insulin is extracted from pork or beef pancreas. Now, highly purified insulins are available, which are less allergenic than previous insulins, and do not cause lipo-atrophy, at the site of repeated injections. The highly purified insulins are now preferred for all new diabetics.

In the UK at present, insulin is available as three strengths (20, 40 and 80 units/ml.), but in the future a single strength of 100 units/ml. may be adopted, as in the USA and some other countries. The type and strength of insulin bottles and cartons is identified by a colour code (20 units/ml. cream; 40 units/ml. blue; 80 units/ml. green). Since there is an ever-increasing number of insulin types available, an identification chart should be available. Insulin should be stored away from sunlight, preferably in a refrigerator, and suspensions should be shaken before use. Soluble insulin is clear, but most longer-acting preparations are turbid.

Routinely, insulin is given subcutaneously. The most popular regimens are twice-daily soluble insulin before breakfast and evening meal, with or without isophane insulin. For emergencies, such as ketoacidosis, or to cover operations, soluble insulin only may be given intramuscularly or by intravenous infusion.

Insulin injection (soluble insulin)
When injected subcutaneously, the maximal effect is from two to six hours, and lasts from eight to twelve hours. For stable diabetics, it is usually necessary to give it twice or thrice daily, either alone, or with longer-acting insulins. Since it is acidic, it cannot be mixed in the syringe with insulin zinc suspensions. In diabetic ketoacidosis, it may be given intramuscularly or by intravenous infusion.

Neutral insulin injection (*Actrapid, Hypurin Neutral,*
Velosulin, Neusulin, Nuso)
These are preparations of soluble insulin which are neutral (and not acidic). Now often used instead of acidic soluble insulin, they can be mixed with insulin zinc suspensions.

Isophane insulin injection (*Hypurin Isophane, Insulatard, Neuphane*)

A combination of insulin with protamine, which prolongs the effect up to 24 hours, when given subcutaneously. Usually given as a twice daily regimen, often with extra soluble insulin to cover mealtimes. It can be readily mixed with soluble insulin; two pre-mixed preparations are available, *Initard* (50% isophane) and *Mixtard* (70% isophane).

Insulin zinc suspension (Amorphous) (*Semilente, Semitard*)

A suspension of insulin with zinc, which has a similar time course of action to isophane insulin.

Biphasic insulin injection (*Rapitard MC*)

A mixture of beef insulin crystals in pork insulin solution. It has a similar duration of effect to isophane.

Insulin zinc suspension (crystalline) (*Ultralente, Ultratard*)

A crystalline suspension of insulin with zinc, to give a duration of action of 24–26 hours.

Insulin zinc suspension (mixed) (*Lente, Lentard, Monotard, Neulente*)

A mixture containing 30% amorphous and 70% crystalline insulin zinc suspension. The peak action is at six hours, and lasts 24 hours. It gives reasonable control with a once-daily injection, if the daily insulin requirements are 40 units or less. However, despite the inconvenience, other twice-daily regimens are often preferred, which give a better control of blood glucose.

Protamine zinc insulin (PZI) (*Hypurin Protamine Zinc*)

This is the oldest available long-acting insulin, and the effect lasts 24 hours or more. Usually given as a single morning

injection together with soluble insulin, PZI contains excess
protamine, which will prolong the action of soluble insulin if
mixed in the syringe. Therefore, a constant technique should
be used.

Oral hypoglycaemic agents

These drugs lower the blood sugar level, but are an alternative
to insulin in mild diabetics only, where the insulin requirement
is low (usually in maturity-onset diabetics). However, they
should not be a substitute for proper dietary management of
obese diabetics. They should not be used for diabetic ketosis.

The sulphonylureas

These drugs stimulate the release of insulin from the pancreas,
and require some functioning pancreatic tissue. Like insulin,
excessive dosage may produce hypoglycaemia and encourage
patients to gain weight. Skin rashes sometimes occur.

Tolbutamide (*Pramidex, Rastinon*)
Dose 0.5–1.5 g daily.

Given as two doses, owing to its rapid effect. May cause
facial flushing after drinking alcohol.

Chlorpropamide (*Diabinese, Melitase*)
Dose up to 500 mg daily.

Since the duration of action may last more than 24 hours, it
is given only once daily. Its elimination is largely renal;
therefore it should be avoided in the elderly and patients with
renal failure, since accumulation will cause prolonged hypoglycaemia. Alcohol-induced facial flushing may occur.

Glibenclamide (*Daonil, Euglucon*)
Dose 2.5–20 mg daily.

Duration of action is usually more than 12 hours. Lower
doses may be given once-daily, but twice-daily is better for

higher doses. It is useful in the elderly since prolonged hypoglycaemia is less likely than with chlorpropamide.

Acetohexamide (*Dimelor*)
Dose 0.25–1.5 g once-daily for lower doses or twice-daily for higher doses.

Glibornuride (*Glutril*)
Dose 12.5–75 mg daily.

Gliclazide (*Diamicron*)
Dose 40–80 mg daily.

Glipizide (*Glibenese, Minodiab*)
Dose 2.5–30 mg daily.

Gliquidone (*Glurenorm*)
Dose 45–180 mg daily.

Glymidine (*Gondafon*)
Dose 0.5–2 g daily.

Tolazamide (*Tolanase*)
Dose 100–1000 mg daily.

The biguanides
These act differently from sulphonylureas, and augment the action of insulin. Anorexia is common, and so they are used in obese diabetics, who are unable to lose weight. Other gastro-intestinal side effects are common. Since phenformin sometimes caused severe lactic acidosis, it is now only rarely prescribed.

Metformin (*Glucophage*)
Dose 1–2 g daily in divided doses.

Gastro-intestinal side effects are not uncommon. It is secreted by the kidneys and should be avoided in renal impairment, since accumulation may cause lactic acidosis. Otherwise, this complication is much less common than with phenformin. It should also be avoided in heart failure and hepatic failure. The risk of side effects is obviously greater in patients taking both a sulphonylurea and metformin, so this combination is now used much less than formerly.

Hyperglycaemic agents

Dextrose injection
Dose 20–50 ml. of a 50% solution.

Hypoglycaemia occurs, owing to a relative excess of insulin, if insulin-dependant diabetics miss meals or undertake unusual exertion. Intravenous 50% dextrose will reverse a hypoglycaemic coma, if adequate oral glucose was not taken prior to loss of consciousness.

Glucagon
Dose 1 mg intramuscularly.

Glucagon is produced by the alpha-cells of the Islets of Langerhans. It raises blood sugar level by causing the liver to release glucose. Glucagon deficiency is unimportant, but glucagon can be given intramuscularly by a nurse or relative to counteract hypoglycaemic coma if intravenous dextrose cannot be given. Higher doses (10 mg) stimulate the heart, and are used in severe beta-blocker poisoning.

Diazoxide (*Eudemine*)
Dose from 5 mg/kg daily in divided doses orally.

Reduces insulin secretion from insulin-secreting tumours, and can be used long-term to prevent hypoglycaemia in such patients. It is of no value in acute hypoglycaemia due to injected insulin.

Adverse effects. These include gastro-intestinal upsets, hypotension, hirsuitism and fluid retention.

PITUITARY GLAND AND HYPOTHALAMUS
Anterior lobe

The anterior pituitary gland produces the two gonadotrophins, namely luteinizing hormone (LH) and follicle-stimulating hormone (FSH), prolactin, thyroid-stimulating hormone (thyrotrophin or TSH), growth hormone (GH) and cortico-trophin (ACTH). There are other peptides produced also, the physiological roles of which are uncertain. The hypo-thalamus increases the secretion of these hormones by gonadotrophin-releasing hormone (LH–RH), and thyro-trophin-releasing hormone (TRH).

These hormones, and synthetic analogues, are used as therapeutic and diagnostic agents.

Clomiphene (*Clomid*)

Dose 50 mg daily for five days.

Increased sex hormones, such as oestrogens, inhibit gonadotrophin release. This action is blocked by clomiphene. By allowing gonadotrophin secretion, clomiphene stimulates ovulation in some cases of secondary amenorrhoea. Un-fortunely, multiple pregnancy may subsequently occur. It is also occasionally useful in certain infertile males.

Adverse effects. These include hot flushes, breast tenderness and nausea.

Chorionic gonadotrophin (*Gonadotraphon L.H., Pregnyl, Profasi*)

Dose 500–5000 units intramuscularly.

Obtained from the urine of pregnant women, and is principally LH. Mainly used as a single injection to treat female infertility, following a course of clomiphene.

Menotrophin (*Gonadotraphon F.S.H., Pergonal*)
This is principally FSH, and is occasionally used with chorionic gonadotrophin.

Gonadotrophin-releasing hormone (LH–RH or gonadorelin)
                              (*Relefact LH–RH, HRF*)
Dose 100 micrograms intravenously.
    Used as a test for suspected hypopituitarism.

Danazol (*Danol*)
Dose 200–800 mg daily orally in divided doses.
    Inhibits pituitary gonadotrophin release, and may be used for endometriosis, mammary dysplasia, and gynaecomastia. May cause mild masculinization, including acne and greasy skin.

Bromocriptine (*Parlodel*)
Dose to suppress lactation, 2.5 mg twice-daily orally.
    By stimulating hypothalamic dopamine receptors, bromo-criptine inhibits the secretion of prolactin and growth hormone. It is used to suppress lactation, to treat infertility and galactorrhoea associated with excess prolactin secretion, and occasionally to treat acromegaly (which is due to growth hormone-secreting pituitary tumours). It is also used in the treatment of Parkinsonism.

Adverse effects. Gastro-intestinal upsets, dizziness and abnormal facial movements (dyskinesia).

Thyrotrophin-releasing hormone (TRH or protirelin)
Dose 40 mg orally or 200 micrograms intravenously as a single dose.
    TRH stimulates pituitary TSH stimulation. Measurement of the TSH response is a good test of thyroid gland function.

Growth hormone (*Crescormon*)
Dose 0.5–1 unit intramuscularly or subcutaneously daily.

Used to treat children with short stature due to growth hormone deficiency. Treatment delayed well after puberty will be ineffective, owing to fusion of bone epiphyses.

Corticotrophin (ACTH) (*Acthar*)
Dose 20–80 units intramuscularly.

ACTH stimulates the adrenal cortex to produce cortisol. Therefore it is used to assess adrenocortical insufficiency, by measuring the plasma cortisol response to ACTH. It has also been used in many conditions as an alternative to synthetic corticosteroids, and is still commonly used in some, such as multiple sclerosis. Since the effect of a single injection only lasts up to six hours, a gel preparation (*Acthar Gel*) is often preferred. It has similar side effects to synthetic corticosteroids, but causes less growth suppression in children. However, it is now used much less, even in children, since this effect is minimal with locally acting steroids (such as inhaled steroids for asthma).

Tetracosactrin (*Synacthen*)
Dose 0.5–1 mg every few days of *Synacthen Depot*.

A synthetic alternative to corticotrophin, with similar effects and side effects. The prolonged action of *Synacthen Depot* means that less frequent injections are required.

Posterior lobe

The posterior lobe of the pituitary gland secretes two hormones: oxytocin, which causes contraction of the uterus in late pregnancy, and vasopressin (antidiuretic hormone or ADH). Oxytocin is discussed in Chapter 19. Vasopressin regulates water conservation by the kidney—deficiency of the hormone results in persistent renal water loss, often ten litres or more daily (pituitary diabetes insipidus). Nephrogenic diabetes insipidus is due to a renal abnormality and will not respond to vasopressin or its analogues: paradoxically, thiazide diuretics are of some value in this condition.

Pituitary (posterior lobe) insufflation (*Di-Sipidin*)
This is used to treat pituitary diabetes insipidus, and is given as snuff, usually three times daily. Since vasopressin is also a powerful vasoconstrictor, great caution must be exercised in vascular disease. It may also precipitate asthma and allergic rhinitis, and cause nasal mucosal degeneration.

Vasopressin (*Pitressin*)
Dose 5–20 units subcutaneously or intramuscularly several times daily.

Occasionally used for diabetes insipidus. Has the same side effects as posterior pituitary extract.

The vasoconstrictor effect sometimes reduces bleeding from oesophageal varices, if 20 units are given slowly intravenously.

Lypressin (*Syntopressin*)
Dose 5–20 units several times daily intranasally.

An analogue of vasopressin available as a nasal spray, but with similar side effects.

Desmopressin (*DDAVP*)
Dose 10–20 micrograms intranasally twice daily, or 2–4 micrograms by a daily intramuscular injection.

Similar to lypressin, but the effects of a single dose last from 12–24 hours.

SEX HORMONES—OVARY

The ovary secrets oestrogens from the Graafian follicle and progestogens from the corpus luteum.

Oestrogens
Physiologically, oestrogens are necessary for the development of female secondary sexual characteristics. They cause hyperplasia of the uterine endometrium, so that sudden

withdrawal causes uterine bleeding (they are occasionally used to produce artificial menstruation).

Oestrogens used therapeutically consist of naturally occurring hormones, together with synthetic analogues. Small doses will inhibit menopausal symptoms, such as hot flushes. They are of benefit in some forms of dysmenorrhoea, by inhibiting ovulation (usually combined with a progestogen). Senile vaginitis and vulvitis respond to local or systemic oestrogens, and they may delay the onset of senile osteoporosis. Some breast cancers respond to oestrogens, as does disseminated prostatic carcinoma. Oestrogens are no longer used to suppress lactation.

Adverse effects. Gastric intolerance, withdrawal bleeding, fluid retention, liver dysfunction. There is an increased risk of thrombo-embolism; and possibly of endometrial carcinoma when given for long periods to post-menopausal women. They are often given for 21 days of a month only, to prevent endometrial hyperplasia. They should be avoided in early pregnancy. In males, they cause gynaecomastia.

Natural oestrogens

Oestradiol
Dose 1–2 mg daily orally (*Progynova* tablets); 1–5 mg at up to two-week intervals intramuscularly (*Benytrone*, oily injection); and 25–100 mg by implantation for longer-term effect.

Oestriol (*Hormonin, Ovestin*)
Dose 250–500 micrograms daily orally.

Conjugated oestrogens (*Premarin*)
Dose 1.25 mg daily orally.
  This is a mixture of equine oestrogens.

Synthetic oestrogens

Ethinyloestradiol (*Lynoral*)
Dose 10–100 micrograms daily.

Stilboestrol
Dose 1–3 mg daily for prostatic cancer, 10–20 mg daily for breast cancer.

Chlorotrianisene (*Tace*)
Dose 12–24 mg daily orally.

Dienoestrol
Dose 0.5–5 mg daily orally.

Piperazine oestrone (*Harmogen*)
Dose 1.5–4.5 mg daily orally.

Quinestradol (*Pentovis*)
Dose 4 mg daily.

Progestogens

The naturally occurring hormone progesterone acts on the uterus sensitized by oestrogens, to facilitate implantation of the fertilized ovum and to decrease uterine motility. Some, e.g. norethisterone, are derived from testosterone, and may cause masculinization of the fetus if used in pregnancy.

Progestogens are used for endometriosis, dysfunctional uterine bleeding and sometimes for uterine carcinoma. Their value in preventing recurrent abortion is doubtful. They are also effective contraceptives in low doses, when oestrogens are contraindicated, but have a higher failure rate than oestrogen/progesterone combinations. They are given daily for this purpose.

Progesterone (*Gestone*)
Dose 5–10 mg daily intramuscularly or 200–400 mg by suppository (*Cyclogest*).
Progesterone has also been incorporated into a sustained-release, intra-uterine contraceptive device (*Progestasert*).

Hydroxyprogesterone hexanoate (*Proluton Depot*)
Dose 250–500 mg weekly intramuscularly.

Medroxyprogesterone acetate (*Provera*)
Dose up to 40 mg daily orally, or 50 mg weekly by intramuscular injection.
It is also used as an intramuscular contraceptive, at a dose of 150 mg every three weeks.

Dydrogesterone (*Duphaston*)
Dose 10 mg twice-daily orally.

Allyloestrenol (*Gestanin*)
Dose 5–15 mg daily orally.

Norethisterone (*Primolut N, Utovlan*)
Dose up to 30 mg daily.
May cause masculinization of the fetus, and acne. The contraceptive dose is 350 micrograms daily (*Micronor, Noriday*).

Ethisterone (*Gestone-Oral*)
Dose 30–50 mg daily orally in divided doses.
May cause virilization as with norethisterone.

Ethynodiol diacetate (*Femulen*)
Dose 500 micrograms daily as a contraceptive.

Levonorgestrel (*Microval, Norgeston*)
Dose 30 micrograms daily as a contraceptive.

Norgestrel (*Neogest***)**
Dose 75 micrograms daily as a contraceptive.

Oestrogen/progestogen combinations

Combinations of oestrogen and a small dose of progestogen are now often used for menstrual disorders, and menopausal symptoms. Similar combinations are widely used as *oral contraceptives*, but often have a lower oestrogen content (20–50 micrograms). The usual oestrogen in these preparations is ethinyloestradiol, and the commonest progestogen is norethisterone.

Oral contraceptives are probably mainly effective by suppressing ovulation, but also reduce sperm motility by altering the consistency of cervical mucus, and prevent implantation of the fertilized ovum.

Adverse effects. Thrombo-embolism is a real risk with oral contraceptives, but overall mobidity and mortality are much less than that associated with pregnancy or abortion. The risk is almost negligible, if a combination with the lowest effective oestrogen content is chosen, but is greater in the presence of other cardiovascular risk factors, especially smoking. Oral contraceptives may cause hypertension, but this usually reverts to normal when treatment is stopped. Weight gain, nausea and headaches are minor side effects, and, rarely, benign liver tumours occur.

With the lower oestrogen preparations, however, there is a greater risk of contraceptive failure, and breakthrough uterine bleeding, especially if tablet taking is haphazard. Concomitant drug therapy may interfere with oral contraception, especially enzyme-inducers, such as rifampicin.

Most oral contraceptives are taken for 21 days, starting on the fifth day of the normal cycle. This is followed by a seven-day interval, during which withdrawal bleeding occurs, before starting the next course. Protection during the first

month is incomplete, but may be improved by starting the contraceptive on the first day of the normal cycle. The regimen with some preparations differs from that above, and so the instructions with each product should be followed carefully.

Combined preparations for menopausal symptoms
Cyclo-Progynova, Menophase, Mixogen, Prempak, Tri-sequens.

Combined preparations for menstrual disorders
Controvlar, Enavid, Metrulen, Norinyl-2, Norlestrin.

Oral contraceptives with 50 micrograms of oestrogen
Anovlar 21, Demulen 50, Eugynon 50, Gynovlar 21, Minilyn, Minovlar, Norinyl, Norlestrin, Orlest 21, Ortho-Novin, Ovran, Ovulen 50.

Oral contraceptives with 35 micrograms of oestrogen
Brevinor, Norimin, Ovysmen.

Oral contraceptives with 30 micrograms of oestrogen
Conova 30, Eugynon 30, Microgynon 30, Ovran 30, Ovranette.

Oral contraceptive with 20 micrograms of oestrogen
Loestrin 20.

Oral contraceptives with a higher mid-cycle oestrogen content
Logynon, Trinordiol.

SEX HORMONES—TESTIS
Androgens

The testes secrete androgens which are responsible for the development of male secondary sexual characteristics. Androgens will inhibit gonadotrophin secretion and suppress

lactation and sperm formation. They also have an anabolic effect on protein metabolism, promoting muscle development, skeletal growth, and prevent osteoporosis.

They are used as replacement therapy in hypogonadal males, but will not stimulate spermatogenesis. They have been used in some cases of breast cancer, but anabolic steroids are now often preferred, since they cause less virilization.

Testosterone
Dose 10–30 mg sublingually daily (*Testoral Sublings*); 10–50 mg of testosterone propionate intramuscularly several times weekly (*Virormone*); 250 mg testosterone enanthate intramuscularly every two weeks (*Primoteston Depot*); 250 mg mixed testosterone esters (oily) monthly (*Sustanon*); 100–600 mg testosterone by implantation every six months.

Methyltestosterone (*Virormone-Oral*)
Dose 30–50 mg daily in divided doses.

Weakly effective by mouth, but often causes cholestatic jaundice.

Fluoxymesterone (*Ultandren*)
Dose 2.5–20 mg daily orally.

A weak androgen.

Mesterolone (*Pro-viron*)
Dose 25 mg four times daily orally.

Androgen antagonist

Cyproterone (*Androcur*)
Dose 50 mg twice-daily orally.

An androgen antagonist used in the treatment of female hirsuitism. Also effective for severe male hypersexuality, but inhibits spermatogenesis.

Anabolic steroids

These drugs retain the anabolic effects of androgens, but cause much less virilization. They are used in some hypoplastic anaemias, and some forms of breast cancer. Although they reduce the itching of cholestatic jaundice, the latter is a common side effect. They should not be used as a tonic, or to increase body weight.

Nandrolone (*Durabolin*)

Dose 25 mg nandrolone phenylpropionate weekly, or 50 mg nandrolone decanoate (*Deca-Durabolin*) every three weeks, intramuscularly.

Norethandrolone (*Nilevar*)

Dose 20–30 mg daily orally.

Methandienone (*Dianabol*)

Dose 5–10 mg daily orally.

Oxymetholone (*Anopolon*)

Dose 5–15 mg daily orally.

Ethyloestrenol (*Orabolin*)

Dose 2–4 mg daily orally.

Stanozolol (*Stromba*)

Dose 5 mg orally daily, or 50 mg every two to three weeks intramuscularly.

13 Drugs used in Anaemia, and Vitamins

IRON

Iron is an important constituent of the haemoglobin of the red blood cell, and of other intracellular oxygen transport proteins and enzymes. Deficiency causes anaemia. Iron-deficiency anaemia may be due to poor diet, hypochlorhydria (following a gastrectomy) or due to increased loss by haemorrhage.

Ferrous salts are usually prescribed since they are better absorbed than ferric salts. Liquid preparations may discolour the teeth. Iron salts cause gastro-intestinal upsets, and so are usually taken after food; they colour the motions black. Iron preparations in the home should be kept secure, since significant poisoning is very serious, especially in children.

Ferrous sulphate is the usual iron preparation. Other, and often more expensive, preparations appear to be better tolerated, only because they contain less absorbable iron.

There is no justification for prescribing compound iron preparations with vitamins, except iron with folate in pregnancy.

Ferrous sulphate (*Feospan, Ferrogradumet*)
Dose 200 mg once to thrice daily.

Ferrous fumarate and ferrous succinate (*Fersamal,*
*Galfer, Ferromyn***)**

Dose 200–600 mg daily.

Ferrous gluconate (*Fergon***)**
Dose 600 mg–1.8 g daily.

Ferrous sulphate mixture, paediatric
Contains 60 mg/5 ml. Well-diluted with water it is useful for
young children. Polysaccharide-iron complexes (e.g. *Niferex*)
or sodium edetate complexes (e.g. *Sytron*) are liquid preparations containing higher concentrations of iron, which,
when diluted, are alternatives to tablets for adults with
dysphagia or gastric intolerance.

Iron dextran injection (*Imferon***)**
Contains 50 mg iron/ml. Dose 1–5 ml. daily by deep
intramuscular injection or the total estimated iron requirement
(average 30 ml.) as a six-hour intravenous infusion in one
litre of dextrose or saline—this should be given very slowly
for the first ten minutes, and the rate subsequently increased
if there is no untoward reaction. The only indication for
parenteral iron is failure of oral iron therapy, owing to poor
compliance, gastro-intestinal side effects, continuing severe
blood loss and resistant malabsorption.

Abscesses may form if the intramuscular injections are not
deep, and the subcutaneous layer should be moved sideways
after penetration prior to entering muscle—the 'Z-shaped'
track prevents the iron-dextran leaking back along the
injection channel, and staining the skin.

Serious anaphylaxis may occur with intravenous iron,
especially in patients with a previous history of allergy—
therefore it should only be used when oral or intramuscular
iron is unsuitable.

Iron sorbitol injection (*Jectafer*)
Dose 2 ml. (100 mg) by deep 'Z-shaped' intramuscular injection (not suitable for intravenous use). Although more rapidly absorbed and better tolerated than iron-dextran, substantial losses of iron may occur in the urine.

DRUGS USED FOR MEGALOBLASTIC ANAEMIA

**Hydroxycobalamin (Vitamin B_{12}) (*Neo-Cytamen,*
Cobalin-H)**
Dose 1 mg intramuscularly every two to three days for two weeks, then 1 mg every two months.

This has largely replaced cyanocobalamin. Deficiency of vitamin B_{12} is usually due to a specific failure to absorb the vitamin (pernicious anaemia), resulting in reduced numbers of red cells, which are large and irregular. Neurological changes can also occur. Replacement with hydroxycobalamin is very effective with an absence of side-effects, but must be life-long.

Folic acid
Dose 5–15 mg orally daily.

Deficiency, owing to malabsorption or poor dietary intake, causes a megaloblastic anaemia with a blood picture similar to that of pernicious anaemia. Although folic acid will improve the anaemia in pernicious anaemia, it worsens the neurological aspects, and must not be given until pernicious anaemia has been excluded or treated.

Small doses are often given prophylactically in pregnancy, and many proprietary iron/folic acid preparations are available for this purpose.

Folinic acid (*Calcium Leucovorin*) is a specific antidote to folic acid antagonists used in malignant disease, such as methotrexate.

VITAMINS

Vitamins are indicated for the treatment or prevention of vitamin deficiency, which only occurs with an extremely inadequate diet.

Vitamin A

This vitamin is present in dairy produce, fish liver oils, and a precursor (carotene) is found in green vegetables and carrots. Deficiency causes night blindness and xerophthalmia.

The dose is 50 000 units daily orally for deficiency (*Ro-A-Vit*); and 4000 units daily as prophylaxis (as Vitamin A and D capsules or halibut liver oil capsules)

Vitamin D

Vitamins A and D are fat soluble, and often found together. Vitamin D is responsible for calcium and phosphorus absorption and laying down bone. Deficiency causes rickets in children and osteomalacia in adults. Deficiency may result from poor diet, malabsorption, lack of sunshine and renal failure. Overdosage causes hypercalcaemia.

Dietary deficiency
Dose 500–5000 units daily.

Available as calcium and vitamin D tablets (500 units/tablet) (*Chocovite*), and calciferol solution (3000 units/ml.).

Resistant rickets and hypoparathyroidism
Dose 50 000–150 000 units daily.

Available as high-strength calciferol (10 000 units/tablet), strong calciferol (50 000 units/tablet), and dihydrotachysterol (500 micrograms–2 mg daily) (*AT 10, Tachyrol*).

Severe bone disease in renal failure
Available as alpha-calcidol (1–3 micrograms daily) (*One-alpha*), and calcitriol (1–3 micrograms daily) (*Rocaltrol*).

B vitamins

Vitamin B is composed of many substances, including hydroxycobalamin and folic acid. Other clinically important B vitamins are thiamine (B_1), riboflavine (B_2), nicotinamide and pyridoxine (B_6), which are often given together to correct deficiency.

Thiamine

Dose 2–5 mg orally daily; if urgent 25–100 mg subcutaneously or intramuscularly initially.

Deficiency (beri-beri) causes heart failure, polyneuritis or encephalopathy, and may be due to protracted severe vomiting, dietary deficiency or alcoholism.

Nicotinic acid

Dose 50–250 mg orally daily.

Deficiency causes pellagra. Nicotinic acid causes vaso-dilatation (often unpleasant) but is occasionally used for this purpose. Nicotinamide does not cause vasodilatation, and is usually preferred when treating pellagra.

Pyridoxine

Dose 50–150 mg orally daily.

Deficiency may occur during isoniazid therapy causing neuropathy and encephalopathy. Some cases of sideroblastic anaemia improve with pyridoxine.

Strong vitamin B compound tablets

These tablets contain nicotinamide (20 mg), pyridoxine (2 mg), riboflavine (2 mg) and thiamine (5 mg).

Parenterovite

A proprietary preparation of vitamins B and C for the emergency treatment of severe deficiencies by intravenous or intramuscular injection.

Vitamin C (ascorbic acid)

Scurvy (vitamin C deficiency) can occur with diets deficient in fresh fruit and vegetables. The dose is 250 mg orally daily in the treatment of scurvy.

Vitamin capsules

Capsules contain vitamin A (2500 units), thiamine (1 mg), riboflavine (500 micrograms), nicotinamide (7.5 mg), ascorbic acid (15 mg) and vitamin D (300 units).

Many proprietary multiple vitamin preparations are available (e.g. *Multivite, Orovite*).

Vitamin K

Vitamin K is essential for the synthesis in the liver of prothrombin and certain other clotting factors; therefore deficiency causes bleeding. This may occur in malabsorption, especially when due to biliary obstruction, since bile salts are essential for the absorption of vitamin K. Deficiency can occur in the newborn, especially if premature, and can be prevented by giving vitamin K to the pregnant mother, or to the baby after delivery (1 mg intramuscularly).

The effect of oral anticoagulants, e.g. warfarin (but not heparin) can be reversed by vitamin K, which is a useful antidote, although the maximal effect may take several hours.

Phytomenadione (*Konakion*)

Dose 5–20 mg orally or intravenously.

Phytomenadione is always effective. There are several synthetic analogues, which are ineffective in some instances (such as reversal of anticoagulation) and are best avoided.

15 Radioactive Isotopes

Atoms are made up of a central nucleus containing a number of positively charged particles called *protons*, with the same number of negatively charged particles, *electrons*, orbiting around them. In addition, the central nucleus also contains *neutrons*.

The atoms of a given *element* all have the same number of protons (the atomic number), but may have different numbers of neutrons. The atomic weight is determined by the number of protons + neutrons. Atoms of the same element (i.e. the same atomic number) which have different atomic weights are called *isotopes*. Most naturally occurring isotopes are stable, but some are not (radioisotopes) and change (decay) into other elements, emitting energy as alpha (α), beta (ß) or gamma (γ) rays (radioactivity). Gamma rays can pass through tissue (like X-rays), but ß rays are absorbed almost totally within the body. Both ß- and γ-radiations are useful medically.

Most medical radioisotopes are not naturally occurring, but are made in either nuclear reactors or cyclotrons.

As radioisotopes emit energy, they decay to non-radioactive elements; the time taken to decay to half their initial radioactivity is the half life. Each radionuclide has a characteristic half life. (the term *radionuclide* is used to denote one specific radioisotope).

In medicine, radioisotopes are used in research, diagnosis and treatment, but only the latter two will be discussed here. Some isotopes will concentrate in a particular organ or group of cells. High radiation doses will result in death of these cells. Lower doses will not damage the organs, but the radiation can be measured by detectors (e.g. a gamma camera), which is useful in diagnosis. Dosage must be carefully controlled to avoid affecting normal cells, which might cause tissue damage, malignant change or genetic damage.

In the interests of safety of patients and staff, all specific instructions regarding the use of isotopes must be obeyed. Extra care must be taken with the higher doses used in treatment.

General rules for handling radioactivity

1. If possible never handle isotopes at all—use forceps or appropriate tongs and equipment.
2. Accomplish the procedure in as short a time as possible.
3. Use shielding to reduce exposure where possible.
4. Use distance to reduce exposure—the dose rate falls off rapidly with distance.
5. Since radiation doses used in diagnosis are very small, there are no special nursing problems. However, care must be taken for several days with the excreta of patients receiving high therapeutic doses, e.g. for thyroid cancer.

Chromium-51 (^{51}Cr) (half life 28 days)
Used commonly to label red blood cells, to measure total body red cell volume, and red cell survival time.

Cobalt-60 (^{60}Co) (half life 5 years)
Very active sources of ^{60}Co are used in industrial sterilization processing of prepacked syringes, needles etc. It is also used in radiotherapy in the treatment of certain tumours. Other radionuclides used in radiotherapy are radium-226, calcium-137 and iridium-192.

Cobalt-57 (^{57}Co) (half life 270 days) **and Cobalt-58** (^{58}Co) (half life 71 days)
Vitamin B_{12} labelled with small amounts of these radioisotopes are used in the diagnosis of pernicious anaemia and other malabsorption syndromes (Schilling test).

Gallium-67 (^{67}Ga) (half life 3 days)
Occasionally used to locate neoplasms or abscesses with the gamma camera.

Iodine-131 (^{131}I) (half life 8 days)
Accumulates in the thyroid gland. Now the treatment of choice for thyrotoxicosis in patients over the age of 40 years, and for thyroid cancer. Lower doses are still occasionally used to assess thyroid function.

Iodine-125 (^{125}I) (half life 60 days)
Human serum albumin labelled with ^{125}I is used to measure total plasma volume and ^{125}I labelled fibrinogen can be used to localize deep venous thrombosis.

Phosphorus-32 (^{32}P) (half life 14 days)
Used to treat primary polycythaemia.

Thallium-201 (^{201}Tl) (half life 3 days)
Occasionally used to detect myocardial ischaemia with the gamma camera.

Technetium-99 (^{99}Tc) (half life 6 hours)
Extensively used with the gamma-camera for scanning brain, liver, lung, spleen and thyroid. A wide range of labelled compounds (i.e. radiopharmaceuticals) have been developed for these tests to enable this radionuclide to localize in the different organs, e.g. phosphate for bone, colloid for liver, macroaggregates for lung.

Xenon-133 (^{133}Xe) (half life 5 days)
An inert gas, which can be inhaled or injected dissolved in saline. Used in lung function tests to assess regional ventilation.

Yttrium-90 (^{90}Y)
This is sometimes implanted into the pituitary fossa for pituitary ablation, for malignant effusions, and occasionally injected into joints severely affected with rheumatoid arthritis.

16 Antibiotics and Chemotherapeutic Agents

Antibiotics are substances produced by fungi and bacteria, although some can be synthesized. They may inhibit the growth of micro-organisms (bacteriostatic) or destroy the organism (bacteriocidal). They can be effective against a wide range of organisms (broad spectrum) or against a limited range of organisms (narrow spectrum). They may be antibacterial, antifungal, or antiviral in action.

Minor infections should not be treated with antibiotics as widespread use in the past has resulted in the development of many resistant strains of micro-organisms. Antibiotics should not be prescribed 'blind', but rather the micro-organism should be cultured in the laboratory and their sensitivity to antibiotics determined. The following factors should be borne in mind when prescribing antibiotics.

The patient

1. Age
2. Renal and hepatic function
3. Antibiotic allergies
4. If female, pregnancy, or taking the contraceptive pill
5. Patient compliance
6. Severity of infection

The drug

1. Identify organism and sensitivity to antibiotics

2. Choose a narrow spectrum antibiotic if possible
3. Avoid combinations of antibiotics (except in tuberculous infections)
4. The dosage and route of administration will depend on the severity of the infection
5. Plasma levels should be the minimum required to counteract the infection
6. The presence of pus or abscesses may inhibit the effectiveness of the drug

The prophylactic use of antibiotics should be avoided except in rheumatic fever, to prevent bacterial endocarditis, and in certain surgical situations.

THE PENICILLINS

Pencillin was the first antibiotic to be discovered. It is extracted from the mould *Penicillium*. Crude penicillin is not a single substance, but a mixture from which a large number of antibiotics have been developed. These include benzylpenicillin (penicillin G), procaine penicillin, benzathine penicillin, benethamine penicillin and phenoxymethylpenicillin (penicillin V).

They are bacteriocidal in action, attaching themselves to the bacteria cell wall causing a weakness and eventual rupture in the developing bacteria. Some bacteria can produce an enzyme called pencillinase which inhibits the effect of penicillin. Fortunately pencillinase resistant penicillins have now been developed (methicillin, flucloxacillin, cloxacillin). Alternatively, a penicillinase inhibitor (clavulanic acid) can be given along with the penicillin.

The penicillin group is relatively non-toxic, while most now are not affected by gastric acid so can be given orally. However, intestinal absorption is poor and many of the penicillins are quickly excreted by the kidneys. High dosages may therefore be necessary. Probenecid prevents the renal excretion of penicillin, so can be given concurrently to produce high plasma concentrations. The penicillins are effective in haemolytic streptococcus infections such as tonsillitis and scarlet fever, endocarditis, meningitis, syphilis, gonorrhoea (although penicillin-resistant strains are now emerging), pneumonia, bronchitis, infective arthritis and osteomyelitis, otitis media, gas gangrene, tetanus and skin infections, such as erisipelas.

Adverse effects. Skin sensitivity to penicillin has been reported and allergic responses can occur.

Benzylpenicillin (penicillin G) (*Crystapen*)
Dose 250 mg intramuscularly four-hourly. Higher doses may be required in pneumococcal meningitis owing to poor transport across the blood brain barrier.

Benzylpenicillin was the first of the penicillins to be used. It is destroyed by gastric acid and so must be given by injection. Once mixed in solution, it must be stored in a refrigerator and used within four to five days.

Procaine penicillin
Dose 300–600 mg intramuscularly once daily.

Procaine penicillin is a compound of procaine and penicillin and is slowly absorbed. It has a delayed effect but a single dose gives adequate blood levels. It is useful in the treatment of syphilis and gonorrhoea.

Benzathine penicillin (*Penidural*)
Dose 450 mg orally six- to eight-hourly, 250 mg–1 g by intramuscular injection.

This preparation is slowly released from the muscle and gives low plasma concentrations up to three weeks after the injection. It is useful in the prophylaxis of rheumatic fever.

Benethamine penicillin (*Triplopen*)
Similar in action and dosage to benzathine penicillin.

Phenoxymethylpenicillin (*Penicillin V*)
Dose 250 mg four- to six-hourly, orally before meals. Available as suspension or syrup.
 This preparation is stable in acid, so can be given by mouth. Since absorption may be unreliable, it should not be used in severe infections.

Phenethicillin (*Broxil*)
Similar in action and dosage to phenoxymethylpenicillin.

Methicillin (*Celbenin*)
Dose 1 g four- to six-hourly by intramuscular or intravenous injection.
 Methicillin was the first of the semi-synthetic penicillins effective against penicillinase producing organisms such as *Staphylococcus aureas*. It is inhibited by gastric acid and so must be given by injection.

Flucloxacillin (*Floxapen*)
Dose 250 mg six-hourly orally or by intramuscular injection.
 Flucloxacillin is more effective than methicillin and can be given orally.

Cloxacillin (*Orbenin*)
Dose 500 mg six-hourly orally in tablet or syrup, or by intramuscular injection.
 Cloxacillin is similar in action to flucloxacillin.

Broad spectrum penicillins

Ampicillin (*Penbritin*)
Dose 250–500 mg six-hourly orally, intramuscularly or

intravenously. Higher dosages may be required in meningitis.

Ampicillin is a broad spectrum antibiotic which is penicillinase sensitive. This renders it ineffective against penicillinase producing staphylococci. It is, however, useful against *Escherichia coli* and *Haemophilus influenzae* and so is effective in chronic bronchitis, urinary infections and otitis media.

Amoxycillin (*Amoxil*)
Dose 250–500 mg six-hourly orally or intramuscularly.

Amoxycillin is similar in action to ampicillin, but is better absorbed.

Pivampicillin (*Pondocillin*)
Dose 500 mg twelve-hourly orally.

Ciclacillin (*Calthor*)
Dose 250–500 mg six-hourly orally.

Talampicillin (*Talpen*)
Dose 250 mg three times daily.

Carbenicillin (*Pyopen*)
Dose 5 g four- to six-hourly by intravenous injection, or infusion.

Carbenicillin is distinguished from other penicillins by its activity against *Pseudomonas* species. Large doses are required, however, preferably by the intravenous route, and it is most effective when combined with gentamicin. It is not absorbed by mouth and is penicillinase sensitive.

Carfecillin (*Uticillin*)
Dose 500 mg–1 g three times daily.

Carfecillin is derived from carbenicillin, but is slowly absorbed when given orally. It is useful in *Pseudomonas* and *Proteus* infections of the urinary tract.

Pivmecillinam (*Selexid*)
Doses: urinary tract infections 200–400 mg orally three to four times daily; salmonellosis 2–4 g daily orally in divided doses.

Pivmecillinam is useful in urinary tract and *Salmonella* infections.

Mecillinam (*Selexidin*)
Dose 5–15 mg/kg six- to eight-hourly by intramuscular or intravenous injection.

This is the active metabolite of pivmecillinam.

Ticarcillin (*Ticar*)
Dose 15–20 g daily.

Similar to carbenicillin, but more effective against *Pseudomonas*.

Mezlocillin (*Baypen*)
Dose 2–5 g intravenously four times daily.

Similar to ampicillin, but has a broader spectrum.

Azlocillin (*Securopen*)
Dose 2–5 g eight-hourly intravenously.

Similar to ticarcillin.

THE CEPHALOSPORINS

The cephalosporins are broad spectrum antibiotics which are useful for gram-positive and for some gram-negative organisms. They are similar in action to penicillin. The cephalosporins are useful in penicillin allergy. Some penicillin-resistant patients will also be resistant to the cephalosporins. Infections caused by *Streptococcus faecalis* and *Pseudomonas aeruginosa* do not respond to the cephalosporins. Many cannot be absorbed when taken orally and so must be given by injection.

Adverse effects. Cephaloridine can cause kidney necrosis which is made worse if the patient is taking frusemide. Hypersensitivity and skin rashes may occur.

Cephaloridine (*Ceporin*)
Dose 500 mg–1 g every eight hours by intramuscular or intravenous injection.

This is now rarely used.

Cephalothin (*Keflin*)
Dose 1 g four-hourly by intravenous injection.

Cephalothin is given for soft-tissue infections and upper respiratory and urinary tract infections. It is less active than cephaloridine, but is less likely to cause renal damage.

Cefuroxime (*Zinacef*)
Dose 750 mg eight-hourly by intramuscular or intravenous injection.

A broad spectrum antibiotic, with some resistance to penicillinase; also effective in gonorrhoea.

Cephradine (*Velosef*)
Dose 250–500 mg six-hourly orally, 500 mg–1 g six-hourly by intramuscular or intravenous injection.

Cephazolin (*Kefzol*)
Dose 500 mg–1 g six-hourly by intramuscular or intravenous injection.

Cephamandole (*Kefadol*)
Dose 500 mg–2 g four- to eight-hourly by intramuscular or intravenous injection.

This has some resistance to penicillinase.

Cephalexin (*Ceporex*)
Dose 250–500 mg six-hourly orally.

Cefaclor (*Distaclor*)
Dose 250 mg eight-hourly orally.

Cefotaxime (*Claforan*)
Dose 1–12 g twelve-hourly by injection.
Similar to cefuroxime, but has some activity against *Pseudomonas*.

Cefoxitin (*Mefoxin*)
Dose 1–2 g eight-hourly by intramuscular or intravenous injection.
Cefoxitin belongs to a group of drugs called cephamycins, which are similar in action to cephalosporins. They are useful in the treatment of peritonitis, but must be given in reduced dosage when renal impairment is present.

THE TETRACYCLINES

The tetracyclines are broad spectrum in action and act by interfering with bacterial RNA activity. They are bacteriostatic in effect against gram-positive cocci and gram-negative bacilli, especially brucellosis. However, their main value now is that they are active against some non-bacterial infections, such as *Rickettsiae, Chlamydia* and *Mycoplasma*. When given orally, however, much of the drug remains within the gastro-intestinal tract. Tetracyclines should preferably be taken with food, although milk and iron, calcium and magnesium salts may reduce absorption. They deteriorate quickly when stored.

Adverse effects. The normal flora of the bowel may be disturbed by unabsorbed tetracyclines, causing glossitis, stomatitis, nausea, vomiting, diarrhoea, pruritus ani. Monilial infections such as *Candida* may be superimposed and bacteria may produce an enterocolitis. Tetracyclines will bind to calcium and cause discolouration of the teeth and inhibition of bone growth in children. Allergic skin rashes can also occur. *Contraindications*. Patients with renal failure and combinations with other antibiotics should be avoided. They should not be given to pregnant women and children.

Chlortetracycline (*Aureomycin*), Tetracycline (*Achromycin*) and Oxytetracycline (*Berkmycen, Terramycin*)
Dose 250 mg six-hourly orally or 100 mg intramuscularly eight-hourly.

Demeclocycline (*Ledermycin*)
Dose 300 mg twelve-hourly.
   Demeclocycline is more efficiently absorbed and so fewer doses are required.

Doxycycline (*Vibramycin*)
Dose 100 mg orally daily.
   Doxycycline is excreted mainly in bile and so does not exacerbate renal failure.

Clomocycline sodium (*Megaclor*)
Dose 170–340 mg orally six-hourly.

Minocycline (*Minocin*)
Dose 200 mg initially, then 100 mg twelve-hourly orally.
   A broad spectrum tetracycline, also effective against *Meningococcus*.

Methacycline (*Rondomycin*)
Dose 150 mg six-hourly orally.

Lymecycline (*Tetralysal*)

THE ERYTHROMYCIN GROUP

Erythromycin (*Erycen, Erythrocin, Ilosene, Retcin*)
Dose 250–500 mg orally six-hourly; 100 mg by intramuscular injection four- to eight-hourly; 300 mg by slow intravenous injection six-hourly.

Erythromycin is effective against a range of bacteria similar to that of penicillin. Toxicity is low and it can be used in the treatment of penicillin-resistant infections and for patients who are sensitive to penicillin. They are also effective in treating Legionnaires disease, *Mycoplasma* and *Campylobacter*. Available as erythromycin stearate, estolate or ethylsuccinate and in capsule, tablet, suspension and injection forms.

Adverse effects. Nausea, vomiting and diarrhoea may occur when large doses are given. Cholestatic jaundice can result with erythromycin estolate.

LINCOMYCINS

Lincomycin (*Lincocin, Mycivin*)
Dose 500 mg six-hourly, 600 mg by injection twelve-hourly.

Lincomycin is useful against gram-positive cocci and penicillin-resistant *Staphylococci*. It penetrates bone easily and so is useful in the treatment of osteomyelitis. Absorption is lessened if taken with food.

Adverse effects. Diarrhoea and severe colitis.

Clindamycin (*Dalacin C*)
Dose 150–300 mg six-hourly orally, 600–2700 mg daily in divided doses by intramuscular injection or slow intravenous infusion.

Clindamycin is a synthetic derivative of lincomycin and is more active and more efficiently absorbed.

THE AMINOGLYCOSIDES

Drugs in this group are effective against a wide range of gram-positive and gram-negative bacteria. Resistance can quickly develop, though, particularly against streptomycin. They are poorly absorbed from the gastro-intestinal tract (unless it is inflamed). Their use is limited by their toxic effects on the ear and kidney. Streptomycin is considered later under anti-tuberculous drugs.

Neomycin (*Nivemycin*)
Dose 1 g orally four-hourly.

Neomycin can be used to sterilize the gut prior to surgery or in acute liver failure. It is not absorbed through the skin or mucosa and so can be used to treat local infections of the skin and eye.

Adverse effects. Damage to the eighth cranial nerve and nephrotoxicity. Hypersensitivity may occur if topical applications are used.

Gentamicin (*Cidomycin, Genticin*)
Dose 6 mg/kg body weight eight-hourly intramuscularly.

This is used in severe infections such as septicaemia and meningitis, and is particularly effective against gram-negative organisms from the urinary tract, e.g. *Escherichia coli, Proteus* and *Pseudomonas*. It is sometimes combined with carbenicillin.

Adverse effects. The possibility of nephrotoxic effects means that creatinine clearance tests should be done, particularly when large doses are used. The dosage should also be adjusted according to the serum gentamicin concentrations, which can be easily measured. Vestibular disturbance may occur.

Kanamycin (*Kannasyn, Kantrex*)
Dose 250 mg intramuscularly six-hourly.
Now largely replaced by gentamicin. Can produce deafness.

Amikacin (*Amikin*)
Dose 15 mg/kg daily by injection.
Amikacin is derived from kanamycin, and is indicated for gram-negative bacteria resistant to gentamicin.

Tobramycin (*Nebcin*)
Dose 3–5 mg/kg body weight daily in divided doses, by injection.
Particularly effective against resistant *Pseudomonas* infections.

Framycetin sulphate (*Soframycin*)
Dose 2–4 g daily orally.
Used by local application in nasal carriers of *Staphylococci.*

Netilmicin (*Netillin*)
Dose 150 mg twice-daily by injection.
Similar to gentamicin, but less toxic.

OTHER ANTIBIOTICS

Chloramphenicol (*Chloromycetin*)
Dose 500 mg six-hourly orally, 1 g six- to eight-hourly by intramuscular injection.
Chloramphenicol is a synthetically produced broad spectrum cheap antibiotic which is effective against *Haemophilus*

influenzae and *Salmonella typhi* and *paratyphoid* organisms.
It is also used in meningitis because of the high penetration of
CSF and in the treatment of conjunctivitis. However, its
severe toxic effects render it only useful in those infections
which do not respond to other antibiotics.

Adverse effects. Chloramphenicol may cause severe bone
marrow depression leading to agranulocytosis, aplastic anaemia
and thrombocytopenic purpura. Peripheral neuritis may also
occur. Premature children may develop the 'grey syndrome'
because of the inability of their liver to conjugate chloramphenicol.

Colistin (*Colomycin*)
Dose 2 million units eight-hourly orally or by injection.
    Colistin is effective against *Pseudomonas* infections. It is
not absorbed from the gastro-intestinal tract.

Adverse effects. It can cause renal and nervous system
damage.

Polymyxin B sulphate (*Aerosporin*)
Dose 500 000 units by intravenous injection.
    Also available as an ointment, or when combined with
neomycin as an aerosol spray (*Polybactrin*).
    Polymyxin is similar to colistin.

Bacitracin
Bacitracin acts against a similar range of organisms as does
penicillin. It is not absorbed from the gastro-intestinal tract
and its toxic effects limit its therapeutic use. It is generally
used as a surface application on the skin, eye, ear or mouth.
Available as an ointment or aerosol spray.

Novobiocin (*Albamycin*)
Dose 150–500 mg orally six- to twelve-hourly.

Novobiocin is used for penicillin-resistant *Staphylococci,* but has severe toxic effects. These include vomiting, diarrhoea, leucopenia, and haemolytic anaemia and skin rashes.

Sodium fusidate (*Fucidin*)
Dose 500 mg orally eight-hourly or by slow intravenous infusion.

It is a narrow spectrum antibiotic which is effective against penicillin-resistant *Staphylococci*, especially in osteomyelitis.

Adverse effects. These include nausea and vomiting, and it is best avoided in pregnancy and hepatic disorders.

Vancomycin (*Vancocin*)
Dose 500 mg six-hourly orally or 1 g twelve-hourly intravenously.

A bacteriocidal antibiotic used in the treatment of antibiotic-induced enterocolitis and to prevent endocarditis. It can cause tissue necrosis and phlebitis and should be avoided in renal impairment.

Spectinomycin (*Trobicin*)
A single dose of 2–4 g by intramuscular injection.

Only indicated for gonorrhoea, if caused by penicillin-resistant organisms, or in patients with penicillin allergy.

THE SULPHONAMIDES

The sulphonamides were first discovered in 1935 from a red dye called prontosil. They are bacteriostatic in action, except co-trimazine and co-trimoxazole which are bacteriocidal. They affect bacterial DNA synthesis by inhibiting folic acid synthesis, and are readily absorbed from the gastro-intestinal tract, reaching peak levels in four hours. They successfully infiltrate most organs, including the placenta. The early sulphonamides are insoluble in acid urine and so may crystallize, causing renal damage. For this reason a high fluid intake of several litres must be taken. Substances which render the urine alkaline, such as potassium citrate or bicarbonate, may help avoid crystallization. They are effective against a wide range of gram-positive cocci and gram-negative bacilli. However, widespread bacterial resistance and the advent of newer, less toxic, antibiotics has reduced their importance. They can generally be given by oral administration, but the sodium salts can be given by intravenous injection. Intramuscular injections can be extremely painful.

Adverse effects. Renal necrosis can occur owing to crystallization. Blood dyscrasias, such as agranulocytosis, aplastic and haemolytic anaemia, and bone marrow depression. Allergic skin reactions such as eczema and rashes occur and sunlight may cause a sensitization reaction. Topical applications may cause a contact sensitivity. Psychiatric illness such as depression have been reported, while gastric upset with nausea, vomiting and diarrhoea can result. *Contraindications:* In pregnancy and premature infants, renal impairment and dehydration. Patients on oral anticoagulants, since the anti-coagulant effect is potentiated.

Sulphapyridine
Dose 1 g daily orally in divided doses.
    This is useful in dermatitis herpetiformis.

Sulphadimidine (*Sulphamezathine*)
Dose 1–1.5 g orally six-hourly, 2 g initially, then 500 mg–1 g eight-hourly by injection.

Sulphathiazole (*Thiazamide*)
Dose 1 g initially, then 1 g four- to six-hourly orally.
    Skin rashes are a common side effect.

Sulphadiazine
Dose 1–1.5 g four-hourly by injection.

Sulphacetamide (*Albucid*)
This is tolerated by mucous membranes, and is used topically in eye infections.

Co-trimoxazole (*Bactrim, Fectrim, Septrin*)
Dose 1 tablet orally six–twelve hourly, 960 mg intramuscularly or by intravenous infusion twelve-hourly.

A newer preparation, containing trimethoprim 80 mg and sulphamethoxazole 400 mg. It is bacteriocidal in action. Trimethoprim also acts by inhibiting folic acid synthesis, required by bacterial DNA. Co-trimoxazole is useful for urinary tract infections, prostatitis, acute episodes of chronic bronchitis, salmonellosis brucellosis and *Pneumocystis* infections. Trimethoprim alone may be equally effective, with fewer side effects.

Co-trimazine (*Coptin*)
Dose 1 tablet orally twelve-hourly.

Largely used in treating urinary tract infections, and contains sulphadiazine 410 mg and trimethoprim 90 mg. Co-trifamole (*Co-Fram*) is similar.

Long-acting sulphonamides
These sulphonamides achieve high plasma levels because of efficient tubular reabsorption. A once-daily dose gives adequate concentrations. The risk of accumulation in the blood stream may make toxic effects more likely.

Sulphadimethoxine (*Madribon*)
Dose 500 mg daily.

Sulphametopyrazine (*Kelfizine W*)
Dose 2 g once a week.

Sulphamethoxypyridazine (*Lederkyn*)
Dose 500 mg daily.
  Can cause severe toxic effects.

Sulphaphenazole (*Orisulf*)
Dose 500 mg daily.

Sulphonamides used in urinary tract infections
These sulphonamides are highly soluble in urine and so the
need for a high fluid intake is less.

Sulphamethizole (*Urolucosil*)
Dose 200 mg orally five times daily.

Sulphafurazole (*Gantrisin*)
Dose 2 g initially, then 1 g four- to six-hourly.

Sulphasomidine
Dose 1–1.5 g orally four-hourly.

Sulphonamides used in intestinal infections
These sulphonamides are poorly absorbed from the gut, so
were used in the past for the treatment of gastro-intestinal
infections and prior to bowel surgery. Because of poor
absorption side effects were less common. They are no longer
recommended for use.

Calcium sulphaloxate (*Enteromide*)
Dose 1 g orally eight-hourly.

Succinylsulphathiazole
Dose up to 20 g daily in divided doses.

Sulphaguanidine
Dose 3 g orally six-hourly.

Phthalylsulphathiazole (*Thalazole*)
Dose 2–12 g daily in divided doses.

NITROFURANS AND OTHER URINARY TRACT ANTIMICROBIALS

The nitrofurans are unrelated to either the sulphonamides or antibiotics. They are bacteriostatic in action, but their mode of action is unknown. They are well absorbed from the gut and are found in high concentrations in the kidneys. This renders them highly suitable for treating urinary tract infections except pyelonephritis.

Adverse effects. Nausea and vomiting can be avoided if taken with food or milk. Peripheral neuropathy and hyper-sensitive reactions can occur. They must not be given in renal failure.

Nitrofurantoin (*Furadantin*)
Dose 100 mg orally six-hourly.

Nitrofurazone (*Furacin*)
Suitable for local application in mixed infections of wounds, burns and otitis externa. If application is prolonged, allergic skin reactions may occur. Can be used for bladder irrigation.

Nalidixic acid (*Negram*)
Dose 1 g orally six-hourly.
 A narrow spectrum drug, useful in *E. coli* and *Proteus* infections of the urinary tract.

Adverse effects. Nausea, vomiting, diarrhoea, neurological disturbance with headaches and convulsions.

Noxythiolin (*Noxyflex*)
Dose: used as a 1–2.5% solution for bladder irrigation.
Effective against bacterial and fungal bladder infections.

Hexamine (*Hiprex, Mandelamine*)
Dose 1 g orally twelve-hourly.
Used for urinary tract infections, but the urine must be rendered acid by addition of ammonium chloride.

Adverse effects. Bladder irritation, dysuria, frequency, haematuria.

Trimethoprim (*Ipral, Syraprim, Trimopan*)
Dose 200 mg orally or by slow intravenous injection.
Trimethoprim is a bacteriostatic drug used in urinary tract infections and in acute and chronic bronchitis. Also useful in malaria prophylaxis (Chapter 23). It acts by inhibiting folic acid synthesis required by the developing bacteria. Combined with sulphonamides as co-trimoxazole and co-trimazine.

Adverse effects. These include nausea, vomiting, skin rashes, pruritus ani and folate deficiency.

Acrosoxacin (*Eradacin*)
A single oral dose of 300 mg is sufficient.
Only used for gonorrhoea in patients allergic to penicillin, or with penicillin-resistant *Gonococci*.

IMIDAZOLE DERIVATIVES

Metronidazole (*Flagyl, Vaginyl*)
Dose 400 mg orally three times daily. Can also be given by infusion, but suppositories are a cheaper alternative.

Therapeutic uses. (1) It is always effective against colonic anaerobic bacteria, e.g. *Bacteroides*, which are important in intra-abdominal sepsis, or other wounds with much necrotic tissue. Also a cheaper alternative to vancomycin for antibiotic-induced enterocolitis. (2) It is effective in the protozoal diseases, trichomoniasis and giardiasis, and higher doses are used for amoebiasis (Chapter 23).

Adverse effects. Gastro-intestinal upsets, peripheral neuropathy with prolonged treatment and causes alcohol intolerance.

ANTITUBERCULOUS DRUGS

The principle governing the treatment of tuberculosis is that the drugs should always be used in combination. Resistant strains of tubercle bacilli can quickly develop if one drug is used alone. In the initial phase of treatment three drugs are recommended. The traditional triad of streptomycin, sodium aminosalicylate and isoniazid is still useful, but rifampicin, ethambutol and isoniazid is preferred. Triple therapy should continue for two to three months, then therapy should continue for another nine to twelve months with a combination of two drugs. The choice of these drugs is determined by the sensitivity of the infecting organisms, the reaction of the patient, and health care funds available. One of the drugs should, however, be isoniazid, combined with perhaps ethambutol or rifampicin. Second-line drugs are available if side effects are severe or if the organisms develop resistance. These include cycloserine, capreomycin, prothionamide and ethionamide.

Streptomycin
Dose 1 g daily intramuscularly. In patients over 40 years of age, lower doses can be given.

A powerful drug that revolutionized the treatment of tuberculosis. It is poorly absorbed from the stomach and, although intramuscular injections can be painful, it is usually given via this route.

Many bacteria, including *Mycobacterium tuberculosis*, quickly become resistant to streptomycin if used alone. Like other aminoglycoides, its excretion depends on renal function, and if this is impaired plasma streptomycin levels should be monitored.

Adverse effects. Vestibular disturbance can result after a few weeks of treatment. The drug should be withdrawn if symptoms of headache, nausea, vomiting and tinnitus occur. Fever and rashes are among the hypersensitivity reactions that appear. Great care should be taken by those handling streptomycin to avoid hypersensitivity.

Isoniazid

Dose 300 mg daily orally or intramuscularly in divided doses.

This is very effective in the treatment of pulmonary tuberculosis and tuberculosis of the genito-urinary tract and meninges, and is widely used. It can be taken orally, but resistance develops quickly if used alone. It is usually combined with streptomycin or rifampicin. Isoniazid can be detected in the urine to check patient compliance.

Adverse effects. In doses of 300 mg daily or less, side effects are few. Insomnia, memory disturbance, poor concentration and occasionally epileptiform seizures occur. Peripheral neuritis may result with high doses, but this can be prevented by the administration of pyridoxine.

Sodium aminosalicylate (*Paramisan*)

Dose 8–15 g daily in divided doses.

Sodium aminosalicylate is the most commonly used form of para-aminosalicylic acid (PAS). It is bacteriostatic in action and must be combined with a bacteriocidal drug, such as isoniazid or streptomycin. It is not effective in tuberculous meningitis. Although cheap, it is used much less now, since more effective drugs are available.

Adverse effects. Gastro-intestinal upsets are common and include nausea, vomiting and diarrhoea. Rarely goitre and psychosis occur. It is given in cachets because of its unpleasant taste.

Rifampicin (*Rifadin, Rimactane*)
Dose 450–600 mg orally once-daily.

This is effective in many bacterial infections, including Legionnaires disease and leprosy as well as tuberculosis. It is given in a single daily dose before breakfast and is often combined with isoniazid (*Rifinah, Rimactazid*) or ethambutol. Unfortunately, its expense limits its usefulness in mass treatment regimens.

Adverse effects. Rifampicin is excreted in the bile and a transient hepatic toxicity with jaundice may occur, with nausea, vomiting and diarrhoea. Allergic reactions such as skin rashes, thrombocytopenia and mild leucopenia are reported. Occasionally fever, dyspnoea and renal failure occur. It reduces the effectiveness of the contraceptive pill and should be avoided in pregnancy. Rifampicin should be used with care in alcoholics and patients with liver damage.

Ethambutol (*Myambutol*)
Dose 500 mg–1 g daily.

Ethambutol is often combined with isoniazid and is still effective even when resistance has developed to that drug.

Adverse effects. It may damage the optic nerve with retrobulbar neuritis, loss of visual acuity and colour vision. Gastritis is a common side effect and it should be avoided in young children and the elderly.

Pyrazinamide (*Zinamide***)**
Dose 500–750 mg orally four times daily.
  Pyrazinamide is derived from nicotinic acid and is useful in the treatment of tuberculous meningitis. It is cheap and rapidly reduces the infectivity of the tuberclea bacilli. Therefore, it is especially valuable in mass treatment programmes. It can cause gastritis, jaundice, fever and urticaria.

Capreomycin (*Capastat***)**
Dose 1 g daily by intramuscular injection.
  It should not be used with streptomycin. Also, it can cause eighth cranial nerve damage, producing tinnitus and vertigo. Hypersensitive reactions and renal damage also occur.

Cycloserine
Dose 500 mg–1 g daily.
  Cycloserine is well-absorbed by mouth and is also used in the treatment of resistant strains of *E. coli* urinary tract infections. High doses may produce drowsiness, headaches, fits and psychosis.

Ethionamide (*Trescatyl***)**
Dose 500 mg–1 g orally daily.

Adverse effects. These include gastro-intestinal disturbance, depression, insomnia and convulsions.

Prothionamide (*Trevintix***)**
Dose 500 mg–1 g daily orally.

ANTIFUNGAL DRUGS

As a general rule antibiotics effective against bacteria have no action against fungi. Most fungal infections affect the skin, and mucous membranes, but systemic infections can also occur. Not all antifungal drugs are antibiotics.

Antifungal antibiotics

The polyene group of antibiotics are derived from *Streptomyces* and are fungicidal in action.

Nystatin (*Nystan*)

Dose 500 000 units–1 000 000 units orally six-hourly.

Nystatin is poorly absorbed from the gastro-intestinal tract, but is effective against local infections, particularly *Candida* (thrush) infections of the mouth, vagina and bowel. Nystatin is available as a mixture, tablets, powder, pessaries and cream. It is too irritant to give by injection.

Adverse effects. It can cause nausea, vomiting and diarrhoea.

Amphotericin B (*Fungilin, Fungizone*)

Dose 250 micrograms–1 mg/kg body weight by slow infusion in 5% dextrose; 200 mg lozenges orally six-hourly for *Candida*.

Amphotericin is not absorbed when given orally, but it can be given by intravenous injection, intrathecally, or applied topically. It is effective against systemic yeast and fungal infections such as histoplasmosis, cryptococcosis, blasto-mycosis and systemic aspergillosis.

Adverse effects. Amphotericin is a particularly toxic drug causing anorexia, nausea, fever, vomiting, tinnitus and kidney damage. Uraemia and hypokalaemia may also occur with parenteral administration.

Natamycin (*Pimafucin*)
Dose 2.5 mg eight-hourly by inhalation, 25 mg tablets per vagina nightly for 21 nights.

Natamycin is prescribed in *Candida* and *Trichomonas* infections of the vagina. It can also be given by inhalation for pulmonary aspergillosis and candidiasis.

Adverse effects. Its side effects include nausea, vomiting and diarrhoea.

Candicidin (*Candeptin*)
Dose 3 mg night and morning for 14 days.

Candicidin is used in vaginal candidiasis. Application is by ointment or tablets, but it can cause local irritation.

The imidazoles
These are a group of recently introduced synthetic drugs.

Clotrimazole (*Canesten*)
Dose 200 mg per vagina for three nights.

Effective in trichomoniasis and candidiasis.

Miconazole (*Daktarin*)
Dose 250 mg orally six-hourly; 200 mg per vagina for seven nights; 600 mg by intravenous infusion every eight hours.

Miconazole is used topically for candidiasis, skin infections, and systemic fungal infections.

Adverse effects. These include local irritation, phlebitis, nausea and vomiting.

Econazole (*Gyno-Pevaryl, Ecostatin*)
Dose 150 mg by vagina for three nights, as cream or pessaries.

Econazole is indicated for candidiasis.

Ketoconazole (*Nizoral*)
Dose 200–400 mg daily orally.
Effective against a wide range of systemic fungal infections.

Miscellaneous antifungal drugs

Griseofulvin
Dose 250–500 mg orally twelve-hourly. Paediatric doses 10 mg/kg body weight daily in divided doses.

Griseofulvin is derived from *Penicillium* moulds. It is well-absorbed from the gut, but ineffective topically. Griseofulvin is effective in widespread ringworm infections of the nails, hair and feet, but may require prolonged treatment. It has few adverse effects but headache, nausea, vomiting and rashes do occur. Absorption is greater if taken with a fatty meal.

Flucytosine (*Alcobon*)
Dose 150–200 mg/kg body weight orally or by intravenous infusion.

Flucytosine is effective against *Candida albicans* and in cryptococcosis. It is well-absorbed from the intestine and is usually given with amphotericin in severe infections, since resistance can develop rapidly.

Adverse effects. There are few, but diarrhoea, vomiting and bone marrow depression do occur.

ANTIVIRAL DRUGS

Only herpes viruses are responsive to drugs, but amantadine (*Symmetrel*) has limited activity against influenza.

Idoxuridine (*Herpid*)
Topical idoxuridine is effective against *Herpes simplex*

infections of the eye, skin and external genitalia, and has
some effect in *Herpes zoster*, if applied sufficiently early in
the illness.

Vidarabine (*Vira-A*)
Dose 10 mg/kg body weight by slow intravenous infusion
daily.

Vidarabine is derived from cytarabine, an anti-leukaemic
drug (see Chapter 18) and both are effective in treating
severe herpes virus infections in patients receiving immuno-
suppressive drugs. Vidarabine may also be effective against
Herpes simplex encephalitis. It can cause gastro-intestinal
disturbances and bone marrow depression, but is less toxic
than cytarabine.

Acyclovir (*Zovirax*)
This has similar indications to those of vidarabine. It is used
topically against *Herpes simplex*.

17 Vaccines, Immunoglobulins and Antigens

Vaccines, containing antigens, give long-lasting protection against certain infectious diseases by stimulating antibody production against the organisms (active immunity). Immunoglobulin preparations contain antibodies and give immediate, but short-lived, protection (passive immunity). Other antigens may be used to detect an antibody response, as a diagnostic test.

If vaccines are not stored and used as recommended by the manufacturer, they may be inactivated.

VACCINES GIVING ACTIVE IMMUNITY

Maximum antibody production in response to vaccination may take several weeks to occur. A greater and more prolonged effect is produced by giving a second vaccination. Booster doses may be required to maintain adequate immunity.

Vaccines are prepared from:

1. Live infectious agents, either harmless but related to the pathogenic agent, or an attenuated form of it. A mild form of the disease is sometimes produced, e.g. following measles vaccine.
2. Inactivated agents. These may produce mild pyrexia and systemic upset.
3. Inactivated toxins produced by an infectious agent (toxoid).

Anthrax vaccine (attenuated)
Dose 0.5 ml. intramuscularly at three-weekly intervals for three doses, then at six months. Reinforcing dose 0.5 ml. intramuscularly.

This is given to persons handling infected skins or infected carcasses and other animal products.

Cholera vaccine (killed)
Dose 0.5 ml. subcutaneously or intramuscularly followed by 1 ml. one to four weeks later. Reinforcing doses six-monthly.

This gives only short-lived and incomplete immunity. It cannot control the spread of the disease.

Diphtheria vaccine, adsorbed (toxoid)
Dose 0.5 ml. intramuscularly. More effective if adsorbed onto aluminium phosphate.

This is usually given to children together with tetanus and pertussis vaccines. A booster dose is only given to adults at high risk of infection, if a Schick test is positive (given as toxoid–antitoxin floccules—*Diphtheria vaccine TAF*).

Other preparations:

Diphtheria and tetanus vaccine (diphtheria and tetanus toxoids**)**

Diphtheria and tetanus vaccine, adsorbed (adsorbed onto aluminium phosphate**)**

Diphtheria, tetanus and pertussis vaccine

Diphtheria, tetanus and pertussis vaccine, adsorbed (commonly used to immunize children**)**

Diphtheria vaccine TAF (contains toxoid–antitoxin floccules**)**

Influenza vaccine (inactivated)
Dose 0.5 ml. intramuscularly yearly during autumn.
 This is recommended yearly for high-risk patients only (e.g. chronic lung disease).

Measles vaccine (live)
Dose 0.5 ml. intramuscularly once only.
 Usually offered to children aged one to two years. May produce a mild measles-like syndrome, or rarely, encephalitis.

Pertussis vaccine
Dose 0.5 ml. intramuscularly or subcutaneously.
 This is usually given combined with diphtheria and tetanus vaccine. Rarely, it produces encephalopathy.

Pneumococcal vaccine
Dose 0.5 ml. intramuscularly or subcutaneously every three years or more.
 Used for splenectomized patients only, who have a high risk of developing pneumococcal pneumonia.

Poliomyelitis vaccine (oral)
Contains three attenuated strains and so must be given in three doses to ensure a good antibody response to each. Rarely it produces a mild polio-like illness, which may affect unvaccinated contacts. Use polio vaccine (inactivated) by intramuscular injection in pregnancy, and patients with diarrhoea or hypogammaglobulinaemia.

Rabies vaccine (inactivated)
This is much safer than earlier vaccines and is offered prophylactically to animal workers at high risk. Effective in infected patients if the course is started within 14 days of the causative bite.

Rubella vaccine (live)
This is offered to pre-pubertal girls aged 11–14 years, to prevent fetal defects, caused by rubella in subsequent pregnancies. Pregnancy is a contraindication, and if women are vaccinated, pregnancy should be avoided for three months.

Smallpox vaccine
Since wild smallpox has been eradicated, the vaccine is now only required for certain laboratory workers and health-care personnel. Eczema, impaired immunity and steroid treatment, are contraindications.

Tetanus vaccine (toxoid)
Three 0.5 ml. doses initially, with reinforcing doses not less than every five years. It is usually combined with diphtheria and pertussis for pre-school children.

Bacillus Calmette-Guérin vaccine (BCG)
Dose 0.1 ml. intracutaneously.

A live attenuated strain of the tuberclea bacillus, offered to all tuberculin-negative children aged 10–13 years, or any tuberculin-negative immigrants from countries with a high incidence of tuberculosis.

Typhoid vaccine
Dose repeated after five weeks.

Contains killed *Salmonella typhi*. Provides 50% protection for up to one year. Vaccines containing *S. paratyphi A* and *B* are probably ineffective for these organisms, and pyrogenic reactions are more likely, but they are still present in the combined vaccines:

Typhoid–paratyphoid A and B and cholera vaccine

Typhoid–paratyphoid A and B and tetanus vaccine

Yellow fever vaccine
One injection of the attenuated strain provides immunity for at least ten years, possibly for life. Avoid during pregnancy and beware of anaphylaxis in persons allergic to eggs.

VACCINATION PROGRAMME

The UK recommendations given in Table 2 may require modification for individuals, or in the event of epidemics, and they do not necessarily apply in other countries.

Table 2. Vaccine programme

Age	Vaccine
Commencing at 3 months	Diphtheria/tetanus/pertussis vaccine with oral poliomyelitis vaccine; Second dose after 6–8 weeks; Third dose after 4–6 months.
During second year	Measles vaccine (live)
Five years or school entry	Diphtheria/tetanus vaccine, and oral poliomyelitis vaccine
11–13 years	BCG if tuberculin-negative, and rubella vaccine (girls only)
15–19 years and school leavers	Tetanus and poliomyelitis vaccine

Vaccination requirements of adults depend on previous vaccination status, and proposed travel to endemic areas (especially cholera, typhoid, yellow fever, poliomyelitis and tetanus).

IMMUNOGLOBULINS GIVING PASSIVE IMMUNITY

Immunoglobulins provide an immediate supply of antibodies to protect the patient. Normal immunoglobulin is prepared for multiple donors. Specific immunoglobulins (rich in antibodies against a particular agent) are prepared from the sera of convalescent patients, or recently immunized donors. Antibodies raised in animals are now rarely used, since anaphylaxis occurs.

Normal human immunoglobulin injection
Adult dose 750 mg intramuscularly.

This is used to prevent hepatitis A (infectious hepatitis) in contacts in institutions, and travellers to high endemic areas. Used in immune deficiency states, and to prevent measles in debilitated children. It is also used in rubella and poliomyelitis.

Antirabies immunoglobulin injection
Dose 20 units/kg intramuscularly and infiltrated around the bite, following exposure to a rabid animal.

Antitetanus immunoglobulin injection
Dose 250 units intramuscularly.

This should be given to unimmunized patients with contaminated or penetrating wounds, in addition to penicillin, wound toilet and a course of tetanus toxoid. Immunized patients only require one booster dose of tetanus toxoid.

Anti-D (Rho) immunoglobulin injection
Dose 150–500 units intramuscularly within 72 hours of childbirth or abortion.

Used to prevent a mother, whose blood group is rhesus-negative, developing anti-D antibodies to the rhesus-positive red blood cells from the fetus, by binding to the antigens on the red cells. If anti-D antibodies develop in the mother, they will cause haemolytic disease in a subsequent rhesus-positive fetus.

Snake anti-venom
This is indicated if significant poisoning follows a snake bite.

The type of anti-venom depends on the snake species—
Zagreb anti-venom is effective for the European adder.
Anaphylaxis may occur, so infusion should be very slow
initially, and adrenaline should be available.

ANTIGENS USED IN DIAGNOSTIC TESTS
Schick test
This is a test used in adults whose occupations put them at
high risk of contacting diphtheria. Schick test toxin (0.2 ml.)
is injected intracutaneously into the forearm. A positive
reading (more than 1 cm redness after 12 hours) indicates
susceptibility to the disease, and necessitates vaccination.

Tuberculin tests
Tuberculin (extracted from tubercle bacilli) is used to assess
the susceptibility to tuberculosis, in children aged 11–13
years, contacts of tuberculosis, and immigrants from high
endemic areas. The Heaf multiple puncture test is a useful
screening test. The Mantoux test is quantitative and 0.1 ml.
of a 1:10 000 dilution of tuberculin is injected intradermally.
A positive test is indicated by a 5 mm or more wheal after 48
hours, and implies a satisfactory immune response. If
negative, the test is repeated with 1:1000, then with 1:100
dilutions.

Kveim test
An extract of sarcoid tissue is injected intracutaneously in
patients with suspected sarcoidosis. Most patients with the
disease will develop a nodular lesion within six weeks which,
on biopsy, confirms sarcoid.

Other infections
Skin tests are occasionally used to confirm past or present
infection in a variety of disorders, including fungal infections,

lymphogranuloma venereum (Frei test) and hydatid cysts (Casoni test).

Asthma

Skin tests using extracts of commonly encountered antigens (such as pollen, house dust mite, cat fur) are sometimes used in the assessment of patients with asthma.

Hay fever

Hay fever is due to allergy to grass pollen. Frequent injections of increasing doses of pollen extract are sometimes given to patients, prior to the hay-fever season, to desensitize them. Although often effective, there is a risk of anaphylaxis occurring following an injection of pollen extract.

18 Drugs Used in Malignant Diseases

Some cancers can be cured, and the aim is to eradicate all neoplastic cells by intensive, and often unpleasant, therapy. However, in many cases, cure is obviously impossible from the outset, and the aim is to suppress the disease, or relieve symptoms. Apart from surgery, radiotherapy and radio-isotopes, drugs that may be used include cytotoxic drugs and hormones.

CYTOTOXIC DRUGS

These act on cellular proliferation. Since tumours have a high cell turnover, they are more susceptible to the lethal effects of the drugs than is normal tissue. However, some normal tissues may also be affected, especially the blood and immune systems, but also the gut, skin, reproductive organs and the embryo. They may also be carcinogenic in the long term.

Combination therapy, with several drugs acting on different stages of cell division, is usually more effective than single drug therapy (e.g. mustine, vincristine, procarbazine and prednisolone for Hodgkin's disease).

Adverse effects. Toxicity is usually reduced and effectiveness increased with high-dose intermittent schedules rather than daily administration. A full blood count should be checked regularly during treatment to avoid serious bone-marrow depression. Especially in leukaemia, the massive breakdown of cells during treatment may cause increased urate excretion and renal calculi, unless prevented by allopurinol. Many of the drugs given intravenously are extremely irritant, and should be handled with care. Cytotoxic drugs are also very expensive.

Alkylating agents
These damage nucleic acids (DNA).

Busulphan (*Myleran*)
Dose 2–10 mg daily; maintenance 1–3 mg daily.

This is used in chronic myeloid leukaemia and sometimes primary polycythaemia.

Adverse effects. May cause gastro-intestinal upset, bone-marrow depression, pulmonary fibrosis, alopecia and sterility.

Chlorambucil (*Leukeran*)
Dose 5–10 mg daily; maintenance 2–4 mg daily orally.

Used long-term alone in chronic lymphoid leukaemia, and with other drugs for Hodgkin's disease.

Adverse effects. Well-tolerated, but can cause bone-marrow depression, convulsions and sterility.

Cyclophosphamide (*Endoxana*)
Dose up to 1.5 g by a single intravenous injection, or 50–100 mg orally as maintenance.

Widely used for haematological malignancies, lymphomas, solid tumours, and sometimes for immunosuppression.

Adverse effects. Causes cystitis unless a high fluid intake is maintained. Lower doses are well-tolerated, but may cause gastro-intestinal upset, alopecia, bone-marrow depression, sterility or pulmonary fibrosis.

Mustine
Dose up to 8 mg as a single intravenous dose.
Often used for Hodgkin's disease.

Adverse effects. Must be used immediately after preparation, and carefully administered into a running intravenous infusion, since it is a strong local irritant. Severe vomiting is common and it may cause bone-marrow depression.

Melphalan (*Alkeran*)
Dose 2–10 mg daily orally.
Given as two- to six-week courses at monthly intervals for myelomatosis.

Adverse effect. Causes delayed bone-marrow depression.

Thiotepa
Dose 45–60 mg into serous cavities.
Mainly used as a single injection in malignant effusions.

Adverse effects. Can cause bone-marrow depression, vomiting and local pain.

Antimetabolites
These interfere with nucleic acid synthesis.

Cytosine arabinoside (Cytarabine) (*Cytosar*)
Dose 2–3 mg/kg daily intravenously for one to three weeks, for acute leukaemia.

Adverse effects. Bone-marrow depression, oral ulceration and liver damage.

Fluorouracil (5-FU)
Dose 12 mg/kg intravenously as part of a daily or weekly

regimen for palliation of breast and some gastro-intestinal and skin cancers.

Adverse effects. Gastro-intestinal upsets, cardiotoxicity, bone-marrow depression, stomatitis, neurological disturbances.

Mercaptopurine (6-MP) (*Puri-Nethol*)
Dose 100–200 mg daily for acute leukaemia; reduce dosage if allopurinol is also given, since this inhibits its metabolism.

Adverse effects. Bone-marrow depression, and liver damage.

Methotrexate
Dose 5–10 mg daily orally for acute leukaemia, choriocarcinoma, and occasionally other tumours. Also given intrathecally for meningeal leukaemia (0.2–0.4 mg/kg). Adjust dosage for impaired renal function.

Adverse effects. Mouth ulcers, hepatotoxicity, bone-marrow depression, renal toxicity and pulmonary infiltrates. Folinic acid (Chapter 14) given subsequently may reduce the toxicity.

Thioguanine (6-TG) (*Lanvis*)
Dose 2 mg/kg daily orally for acute leukaemia, reduced in renal failure.

Adverse effect. Bone-marrow depression.

Azathioprine (*Imuran*)
Dose 1–5 mg/kg daily.
    Used clinically as an immunosuppressant, to prevent transplant rejection, and in auto-immune and collagen diseases, which have not responded adequately to corticosteroids.

Adverse effects. Usually well-tolerated, but may cause bone-marrow depression, and since it is converted to mercaptopurine, the dosage should be reduced if allopurinol is also given.

Cytotoxic antibiotics

These interfere with ribonucleic acid (RNA) replication and protein synthesis.

Actinomycin D (*Cosmegen Lyovac*)

Dose 15 micrograms/kg intravenously daily, as a bolus in a running drip, since it is a local irritant.

Mainly used for childhood tumours.

Adverse effects. May cause bone-marrow depression and mouth ulceration.

Bleomycin

Dose 20 units/week intravenously or intramuscularly.

Used in some carcinomas and lymphomas.

Adverse effects. Causes anaphylaxis, progressive pulmonary fibrosis and skin reactions.

Daunorubicin (daunomycin)

Dose 1 mg/kg daily intravenously for acute leukaemia.

Adverse effects. Causes bone-marrow depression and cardiotoxicity. Colours urine red.

Doxorubicin (*Adriamycin*)

Dose 60–90 mg/m^2, through a running intravenous infusion for acute leukaemia and other tumours.

Adverse effects. Local irritant (care when handling) and causes bone-marrow depression and cardiotoxicity. Produces red urine.

Mithramycin (*Mithracin*)
Dose 25–50 micrograms/kg intravenously on alternate days.
  Not used except for the emergency treatment of severe hypercalcaemia.

Adverse effects. Causes severe bone-marrow depression and haemorrhage.

Vinca alkaloids
These are extracted from the plant *Vinca rosea*. They inhibit cell division.

Vinblastine (*Velbe*)
Dose 0.1–0.15 mg/kg intravenously weekly for lymphomas.

Adverse effects. Causes bone-marrow suppression, local irritation (care when handling), mouth ulceration and peripheral neuropathy.

Vincristine (*Oncovin*)
Dose 0.5–1.5 mg/m² for lymphomas and leukaemia.

Adverse effects. More likely than vinblastine to cause peripheral neuropathy, but haematological effects are less severe.

Other cytotoxic drugs

Asparaginase (colaspase) (*Crasnitin*)
Dose 10–500 units/kg daily intravenously for leukaemia.

Adverse effects. Toxicity frequent, especially hepatic, and may cause anaphylaxis.

Carmustine (BCNU)
Dose 75–100 mg/m² intravenously for two doses only, to be repeated after two months, owing to delayed effect on bone marrow. Used for brain tumours and Hodgkin's disease. Lomustine (CCNU) is a similar drug.

Cisplatin (*Neoplatin*)
This is active against many tumours.

Adverse effects. May cause deafness and renal damage, as well as bone-marrow depression. Maintain adequate fluid intake and reduce dose if there is renal failure.

Dacarbazine (DTIC)
Total dose 1 gm/m² intravenously for Hodgkin's disease and malignant melanoma.

Adverse effects. Local irritant, and causes severe nausea and vomiting, bone-marrow depression, and hepatic and renal toxicity.

Hydroxyurea (*Hydrea*)
Dose 25 mg/kg daily as a second-choice drug for chronic myeloid leukaemia.

Adverse effect. Causes bone-marrow depression.

Procarbazine (*Natulan*)
Dose 50–300 mg daily for Hodgkin's disease.

Adverse effects. Potentiates sedatives and hypnotics, produces an unpleasant reaction with alcohol (like disulfiram) and is a weak monoamine oxidase inhibitor. Therefore, avoid alcohol, sympathomimetic drugs, and foods containing tyramine (e.g. cheese).

Razoxane (*Razoxin***)**
Dose 125 mg twice-daily.
    May increase tumour sensitivity to radiotherapy.

HORMONES

Stilboestrol
This is an oestrogen, used for symptomatic relief in disseminated prostatic carcinoma (1 mg daily). It is occasionally
used for post-menopausal breast cancer (15 mg daily), but
may also cause hypercalcaemia.
    Other oestrogens used in malignant disease include ethinyl-
oestradiol, chlorotrianisene, fosfestrol and polyestradiol.

Adverse effects. Vomiting, fluid retention, loss of libido and
gynaecomastia.

Tamoxifen (***Nolvadex***)
Dose 10–20 mg twice-daily.
    Blocks oestrogen receptors in breast cancer.

Adverse effects. Usually well-tolerated, but may precipitate
menopausal symptoms and hypercalcaemia.

Hydroxyprogesterone
A progestogen, dose 1 g weekly intramuscularly, mainly for
breast cancer.
    Similar progestogens include gestronol, medroxyprogesterone
and norethisterone.

Adverse effects. Hepatotoxicity and hypercalcaemia occur.

Fluoxymesterone
An anabolic steroid, used for pre-menopausal breast cancer
(30 mg daily orally).

Similar drugs are nandrolone and drostanolone.

Adverse effects. May cause hepatotoxicity, masculinization, fluid retention and hypercalcaemia.

Corticosteroids

Prednisolone and prednisone (in combination with cytotoxic drugs) are used for lymphomas, leukaemia and certain other tumours (see Chapter 13).

19 Drugs Used in Midwifery

Medicines and controlled drugs are of extreme importance in child-bearing as they may affect not only the mother but also her unborn child. The earlier in pregnancy the medicine is taken, the more severe is the effect on the fetus. In some pregnancies the embryo may suffer gross damage or even death as a result of drugs taken by the mother. Examples of harmful drugs are tetracycline, cytotoxic drugs, aspirin and oestrogens. Drugs may also affect the neonate during breast feeding by passing from the mother's blood to the milk.

The midwife is permitted to obtain and administer on her own responsibility certain Prescription Only Medicines (POM) such as dichloralphenazone, pentazocaine, promazine, syntometrine, lignocaine and naloxone (Statutory Instrument 2127—The Medicine Prescription Only Order 1977). A practising midwife shall not administer an inhalational analgesic, unless she has received approved instruction and a registered medical practitioner has signed a certificate stating that there is no contraindication to the administration of the analgesic.

Midwives who are instructed in the technique of 'topping-up' epidural analgesia and have received approval from the responsible doctor can administer maintenance doses of the analgesic.

Analgesics

Pethidine
Dose 100–200 mg intramuscularly.

Pethidine is a narcotic analgesic and antispasmotic; it is the most widely used analgesic in the obstetric field, relieving the pain of labour without diminishing the force of uterine contraction. Because pethidine crosses the placental barrier it may cause neonatal respiratory depression. However, this can be reversed with naloxone (Narcan) (Chapter 8). The Misuse of Drugs (Amendment) Regulation 1974 permits midwives who have notified their intention to practise, to possess and administer pethidine so far as is necessary in the practice of their profession.

Pentazocine (*Fortral*)
Dose 30–40 mg intramuscularly.
Pentazocine is a powerful analgesic which is almost free from addictive properties. It has effects similar to those of pethidine.

Naloxone (*Narcan*)
Dose 10 micrograms/kg body weight.
Naloxone is a selective narcotic antagonist reversing, complete or partial, narcotic depression including respiratory depression.

Promazine (*Sparine*)
Dose 25–50 mg intramuscularly.
This drug may be given to potentiate pethidine, to relieve anxiety and for its anti-emetic properties.

Inhalational analgesia

Nitrous oxide and oxygen (*Entonox*)
These gasses are prepared in a single cylinder containing 50% of each. This concentration is approved by the Central Midwives Board. It is most effective in the latter part of the first stage of labour and during the second stage. It does not

reduce the maternal oxygen intake and so does not predispose
to fetal hypoxia.

Methoxyflurane (*Penthrane*)
The Central Midwives Board approves the use of a concentration in air of 0.35% given in the Cardiff Inhaler.

Epidural analgesia
Epidural analgesics can give complete relief from pain in
labour without causing respiratory depression of the fetus.
Midwives are permitted to administer 'topping-up' of the
analgesic if given instructions and approval to do so (see
above).

Before each 'top-up' dose, blood pressure, pulse and fetal
heart rate should be taken and these measurements repeated
at five to ten minute intervals for thirty minutes after
administration.

Bupivacaine (*Marcain Plain*)
Dose 8–16 ml. of 0.25% concentration, 4–8 ml. of 0.5%
concentration.

Bupivacaine is preferred to lignocaine because its length of
action is considerably greater and it is just as effective,
without adrenaline being added.

Lignocaine (*Lidothesin, Xylocaine*)
Dose 15–20 ml. of 1.5% concentration with 1/200 000
adrenaline.

Anticonvulsants

Chlormethiazole (*Heminevrin*)
Dose 0.8% by intravenous infusion.

This drug is a hypnotic and anticonvulsant. It may be used
in pre-eclampsia and eclampsia.

Diazepam (*Valium*)
Dose 30 mg intravenously.

Diazepam is used in the treatment of convulsions in pre-eclampsia. However, it may be responsible for hypotonia and jaundice in the neonate.

Oxytocic preparations
These are substances named after the first member of the group oxytocin, a hormone secreted by the posterior pituitary gland which causes the uterus to contract.

Oxytocin (*Syntocinon*)
Dose 0.5 units in 540 ml. glucose increasing to 2.5 units.

This preparation is given to induce or accelerate labour. It may cause fetal hypoxia or anoxia.

Oxytocin may also be used as a nasal spray for the mother two to five minutes before the baby is put to the breast to relieve engorgement of the breasts.

Ergometrine
Dose 125–250 mg intravenously.

Although not related to oxytocin, it causes uterine contraction, and is given to control haemorrhage, both post-partum and after abortion. *Syntometrine* (ergometrine 500 micrograms with oxytocin 5 units) is a proprietary preparation, commonly given intramuscularly at delivery to prevent postpartum haemorrhage.

Prostaglandins
These are naturally occurring hormones, given to induce pre-term labour (e.g. if intra-uterine death) or induce abortion. They are given by intravenous infusion, and sometimes by extra- or intra-amniotic infusion. Adverse effects are dose-related.

Dinoprost (*Prostin F2 alpha*)
Dose 2.5–25 micrograms/min by intravenous infusion.

Dinoprostone (*Prostin E2*)
Dose 0.25–5 micrograms/min by infusion. Can also be given orally (500 micrograms hourly).

20 Drugs Used in Paediatrics

Almost all drugs given to an adult may be given to a child, though the dose is adjusted according to certain criteria. Certain drugs should be avoided, e.g. tetracyclines, which discolour developing teeth. They may also be flavoured or coloured to encourage the child to take the medicine. Unfortunately, liquid preparations contain high sugar concentrations which encourage dental caries.

The criteria have been incorporated into formulae for calculation of drugs dosage.

CLARKE'S RULE

$$\text{Child's dose} = \frac{\text{adult dose} \times \text{child's weight in kg}}{70}$$

Example
Dose for a child of 7 years weighing 22.5 kg.
Adult dose is 200 mg.

$$\text{Child's dose} = \frac{200 \times 22.5}{70} = 64 \text{ mg}$$

YOUNG'S RULE

$$\text{Child's dose} = \frac{\text{adult dose} \times \text{child's age}}{\text{child's age} + 12}$$

Example
Dose for a child of 7 years.
Adult dose is 200 mg.
Child's dose $= \dfrac{200 \times 7}{7 + 12} = 73$ mg

PERCENTAGE METHOD

Child's dose $= \dfrac{\text{surface area of child} \times \text{adult dose}}{\text{surface area of adult}}$

Example
Dose for a child of 7 years of average height and weight.
Child's dose $= \dfrac{0.85}{1.7} = \dfrac{1}{2}$ or 50% of the adult dose.

The surface area is estimated from weight and height or weight alone. It is measured in square metres (m^2) and read from a surface-area nomogram.

PHARMACOKINETICS

Apart from neonates, children cope with drugs, and eliminate them by hepatic metabolism or renal excretion, as efficiently, if not more so, than adults (children are 'little adults'). However, in babies less than one month old these mechanisms are not fully developed, and excess dosage should be carefully avoided.

Medicines should not be mixed with feeds, which might impair their absorption.

21 Drugs Acting on the Eye, Ear, Nose and Throat

EYE

Preparations acting on the eye include lotions, ointments, drops and sub-conjunctival injections.

Lotions are used to remove foreign material from the eye.

Ointments are applied to the lid margins in blepharitis or in conjunctival fornices to affect the eye itself. They may be used to prevent adhesion of lids or adhesion of lids to eye.

Drops may be used to dilate or constrict the pupil, to provide anaesthesia or as a means of overcoming infection. Eye drops can be prepared as aqueous or oily solutions; the oily ones are the longer acting. To avoid bacterial contamination, single-application containers should be used where possible. Multiple application preparations with preservative should be discarded after a month.

Sub-conjunctival injections are used in the treatment of acute intra-ocular infection. Prior to injection anaesthetic drug drops are instilled.

Irrigating fluids

Sodium bicarbonate
Concentration 3.5%.

This solution is useful in removing grease from lids and lashes. It is also used to irrigate the eye after acid burns.

Sodium chloride
Concentration 0.9%.

Drugs which dilate pupils (mydriatics)

Atropine
Concentration 1.0% atropine sulphate.
   Atropine causes dilation of the pupil and paralysis of accommodation. The effect lasts several days and this rests the eye, thus reducing inflammation.

Therapeutic uses. Used to facilitate examination of the eye, in the treatment of iritis and following certain eye injuries and operations.

Adverse effects. In the older person there is a danger of precipitating an attack of glaucoma, which can lead to blindness. Atropine may also cause local skin reaction.

Homatropine
Concentration 2.0% homatropine hydrobromide.
   Its action is similar to that of atropine, though with a more rapid onset and shorter effect. Its effects can be reversed by pilocarpine.

Adrenaline (*Epifrin, Eppy, Simplene*)
Concentration 1.0%.

Therapeutic uses. Adrenaline reduces conjunctival congestion and may lower intra-ocular tension. It has little effect on accommodation.

Lachesine
Concentration 1.0% lachesine chloride.

Cyclopentolate (*Mydrilate*)
Concentration 0.5% or 1.0% cyclopentolate hydrochloride.
   Its action is more rapid in onset and shorter in effect than that of atropine.

Phenylephrine (*Isopto Frin, Prefrin, Zincfrin*)
   This drug is used to lower intra-ocular pressure in acute glaucoma. It has little effect on accommodation.

Tropicamide (*Mydriacyl*)
0.5% and 1%.
   The shortest-acting mydriatic.

Drugs which constrict pupils (miotics)

Physostigmine (*Eserine*)
Concentration 0.25% physostigmine sulphate.
   Used in the treatment of glaucoma. Contraction of pupils facilitates drainage.

Pilocarpine (*Minims Philocarpine Nitrate*)
Concentration 1.0% pilocarpine hydrochloride.
   Pilocarpine is used in the long-term treatment of glaucoma, and to reverse the effect of mydriatics.

Ecothiopate (*Phospholine Iodide*)
Concentrations 0.06%, 0.125% and 0.25% ecothiopate iodide.

Other drugs used in the treatment of glaucoma

(a) Eye Drops
1. Miotics, e.g. pilocarpine

2. Adrenaline, phenylephrine, guanethidine (*Ganda, Ismelin*)
3. Beta-blockers, e.g. timolol (*Timoptol*)

(b) Carbonic Anhydrase Inhibitors

Acetazolamide (*Diamox*)
Dose 250 mg six-hourly or 'sustets' 500 mg twice-daily.

Dichlorphenamide (*Daranide, Oratrol*)
Dose 100 mg twice-daily.

Anaesthetics used in the eye

After an anaesthetic is used, an application of oil or ointment is advisable as a protection against foreign bodies.

Cocaine
Concentration up to 5.0% cocaine hydrochloride.

Cocaine causes local anaesthesia and dilation of the pupil. The effect lasts several hours. On administration it causes severe stinging. A more long-term side effect may be clouding of the cornea.

Amethocaine
Concentration 0.5% or 1.0% amethocaine hydrochloride.

Amethocaine is used in the removal of foreign bodies. It does not dilate the pupils or dry the cornea and its effects last for half to one hour. It causes severe stinging on administration.

Oxbuprocaine (*Benzoxinate*)
Its onset is rapid and its effects short. It does not cause as severe stinging as cocaine or amethocaine.

Proxymetacaine (*Ophthaine*)
Concentration 0.5% proxymetacaine hydrochloride.

This drug is used in routine tonometry.

Antibiotics used in the eye

Treatment, if possible, should be delayed until the sensitivity
of the organism is determined. Many severe infections can be
cleared within a few hours of administration, and prolonged
use should be avoided. Local hypersensitivity to antibiotics
may occur.

Chloramphenicol (*Chloromycetin*)
Usual concentration 0.5% in drops, 1.0% in ointment.

Neomycin (*Graneodin, Myciguent, Neosporin, Nivemycin*)
Usual concentration 0.5% in drops and ointment.

Sulphacetamide (*Albucid, Ocusol*)
Usual concentration 10.0% in drops, 6.0% in ointment.

Framycetin (*Framygen, Sotramycin*)
Usual concentration 0.5% eyedrops or ointment.

Polymyxin (*Neosporin, Polyfax*)

Gentamicin (*Alcomicin, Genticin*)
Usual concentration 0.3% eye drops, only for pseudomonas.

Tetracycline (*Achromycin*)
Usual concentration 1% ointment is used for trachoma.

Idoxuridine (*Dendrid, Idoxene, Kerecid, Ophthalmedine*)
Usual concentration 0.1% in drops, 0.5% in ointment.
   Idoxuridine is an antiviral agent which inhibits viral DNA
production. It is used in the treatment of denritic keratitis due
to *Herpes simplex*. Treatment using drops is hourly during
the day and two-hourly at night. When using ointment,
administration is less frequent. Prolonged use may damage
the cornea. Vidarabine (*Vira-A*) is a recent alternative.

Corticosteroids

These are only indicated for certain non-infective inflammatory conditions, e.g. iritis. Glaucoma may be precipitated. If used inappropriately for infections, such as dendritic ulcers due to *Herpes simplex*, these will be exacerbated.

Hydrocortisone (*Hydrocortistab*)

Prednisolone (*Predsol*)

Betamethasone (*Betnesol*)

Dexamethasone (*Maxidex*)

Miscellaneous preparations

Fluorescein
Usual concentration 1.0%.

Fluorescein is a dye which, when instilled into the eye and then washed out with normal saline, will leave a greenish stain on ulcers and abrasions of the cornea. An intravenous form is used to show leakage from retinal blood vessels.

Hypromellose (*Isopto Plain, Adsorbotear, Tears Naturale*)
Used for chronic 'dry eyes' due to tear deficiency, as occurs sometimes in rheumatoid arthritis.

TOPICAL DRUGS ACTING ON THE EAR

Aluminium acetate
Usual concentration 13.0%.

Aluminium acetate as drops or impregnating a gauze pack may be used in the treatment of otitis externa. With prolonged use concretions may form in the meatus.

Sodium bicarbonate
Usual concentration 5.0%.

Sodium bicarbonate facilitates the removal of wax from the ear. Glycerol and warm olive oil may also be used.

Corticosteroid ear drops
These are used for eczematous otitis externa.

Hydrocortisone (*Hydrocortistab*)

Prednisolone (*Predsol*)

Betamethasone (*Betnesol*)

Antibacterial ear drops
These are occasionally used for infected eczema. Local hypersensitivity may occur and prolonged use may cause bacterial resistance or fungal infection. Chloramphenicol, framycetin, gentamicin, neomycin, nitrofurazone and tetracycline are available.

Combinations with hydrocortisone are popular (e.g. *Otosporin*).

DRUGS ACTING ON THE NOSE

Preparations instilled into the nose have a very transient action as the cilia will have moved them in less than twenty minutes. Preparations that inhibit ciliary action include oily preparations, which may pass into the trachea during sleep causing pneumonia, and those with a strong solution of antibiotics or vasoconstrictors that may impede the clearance of material from the nasal cavities.

Ephedrine
Usual concentration is ephedrine 0.5% with chlorbutol 0.5%.

Ephedrine is a vasoconstrictor and causes shrinkage of the swollen mucus membrane giving temporary relief to nasal congestion and aiding drainage from infected nasal sinuses. Unfortunately, tolerance rapidly develops, the nasal cilia are damaged and rebound congestion occurs when treatment is stopped.

Phenylephrine, xylometazoline (*Otrivine*) and oxymeta-zoline (*Afrazine*) are similar.

Sodium cromoglycate insufflation (*Rynacrom*)

Dose 10 mg into each nostril four times daily.

This drug is used in the prophylactic treatment of allergic rhinitis. It acts by blocking the last stage of the allergic reaction, so preventing the release of substances that provoke sneezing, mucosal congestion, and excess mucous production.

Corticosteroid sprays are also used.

DRUGS ACTING ON THE MOUTH AND THROAT

Sodium bicarbonate or sodium chloride solutions are used as mouth washes.

Compound thymol glycerin

Dilute one part to three parts water.

Used as a mouth wash.

Chlorhexidine (*Corsodyl, Eludril*)

A mouth wash, which may reduce plaque formation.

Nystatin mixture (*Nystan*)

Dose 1 ml. four times daily as a mouth wash.

Nystatin is a fungistatic used in the treatment of *Candida* (thrush). Amphotericin (*Fungilin*) lozenges are an alternative. If these fail, miconazole (*Daktarin*) gel may be effective.

Iodine compound paint
Concentration 1.2% iodine (Mandl's paint) or 2.5% potassium
iodine in glycerin.

Used for oral ulceration, such as *Herpes* or *Candida*.
Crystal violet is similarly used, especially in children.

Aphthous ulcers
Many preparations for treatment are available, which should
be kept in contact with the ulcer.

Carboxymethylcellulose (*Orabase, Orahesive*)

Corticosteroids (*Adcortyl, Corlan*)

Carbenoxolone (*Bioral*)

Tetracycline

Choline salicylate (*Bonjela, Teejel*)

Local anaesthetics (e.g. benzocaine) (*Oral-B*)

22 Local Applications and Antiseptics

Topical preparations (applied to the skin) usually consist of an active drug in a base or vehicle.

Absorption

The rate of absorption depends on the temperature and the concentration of the drug. It also depends on the condition of the skin—where the skin is inflamed, for example with psoriasis, absorption is more rapid. Where the keratin layer is thicker, for example on the palms of the hands, absorption is slower.

Absorption is enhanced by occlusion, which has the effect of softening the keratin layer. However, there is the danger of causing secondary infection using this method.

Vehicle (base)

The active drug is contained either dissolved or suspended in a cream, ointment, lotion or paste.

Cream

These are emulsions, either oil in water or water in oil. Evaporation of water cools the skin. The oily compound acts as a barrier for water, preventing passage both to and from the skin.

Therapeutic uses. For dry skin, by preventing loss of moisture, or as a protection against external moisture, e.g. wet nappies.

Ointments
These have an oil or grease base.

Therapeutic uses. Principally in the treatment of chronic dry-skin disorders.

Shake lotion
An aqueous suspension of insoluble powder.

Therapeutic uses. A soothing effect and gives relief of pruritis. Used to cool and dry inflamed and weeping areas of skin, e.g. calamine lotion.

Pastes
Ointments containing insoluble powder.

Therapeutic uses. Applied to inflamed or excoriated skin. Absorbs secretions and does not cause heat retention.

ACTIVE AGENTS
Antibacterial
Where possible antibiotics that can be used systemically should not be used topically, to avoid the risk of skin sensitivity developing, which is more likely to occur in topical application. Their widespread use will also encourage the proliferation of organisms with antibiotic resistance. Some are available as aerosol sprays. Therefore antibiotics not available for systemic use (e.g. polymixin) are preferred. Established infections are often best treated with systemic antibiotics.

Chloramphenicol cream (1%)

Framycetin (*Framygen, Soframycin, Sofra-Tulle***)**

Fusidic acid (2%) (*Fucidin*)

Gentamicin (0.3%) (*Cidomycin, Genticin*)

Mafenide (8.5%) (*Sulfamylon*)
Used for *Pseudomonas* infection of burns.

Neomycin (*Myciguent, Nivemycin*)
Also available mixed with other antibiotics, e.g. *Cicatrin, Polybactrin.*

Nitrofurazone (*Furacin*)

Polymixin B

Polynoxylin (*Anaflex, Ponoxylan*)

Silver sulphadiazine (1%) (*Flamazine*)
Popular for *Pseudomonas* infections in burns. Antibiotic resistance has not yet been a problem.

Tetracyclines (*Achromycin, Aureomycin, Terramycin*)

Triclocarban (*Cutisan*)

Antifungal

Benzoic acid compound ointment (Whitfield's ointment)
Used for ringworm and *Tinea Pedis* (athletes' foot).

Zinc undecenoate ointment (*Mycota, Tineafax*)
Used for *Tinea Pedis*.

Amphotericin (3%) (*Fungilin*)
Used for *Candida* infections.

Chlorphenesin (1%) (*Mycil*)

Clotrimazole (1%) (*Canesten*)
Used for ringworm, and *Candida*.

Econazole (1%) (*Ecostatin, Pevaryl*)

Miconazole (2%) (*Daktarin, Dermonistat*)
Miconazole and econazole are similar to clotrimazole.

Natamycin (2%) (*Pimafucin*)

Nystatin (*Multilind, Nystan*)
Used for *Candida* infections.

Pecilocin (*Variotin*)

Tolnaftate (1%) (*Tinaderm*)

Antiparasitic

Benzyl benzoate (*Ascabiol*)
Used for scabies. Applied to all the family over whole body
with brush and repeated the following day.

Crotamiton (*Eurax*)
Used for scabies. It also has antipruritic properties.

Gamma benzene hexachloride (*Lorexane, Quellada*)
Used for lice and scabies in children.

Carbaryl (*Carylderm, Derbac Shampoo*)
A shampoo or lotion for head lice.

Malathion (*Prioderm, Derbac Liquid*)
An alternative to carbaryl.

Monosulfiram (*Tetmosol*)
Effective for scabies, lice and other parasites. The lotion should be diluted with water prior to application.

Antiviral

Idoxuridine (*Herpid, Iduridin*)
Available as a 5% solution in dimethyl sulphoxide. Effective if applied during the first few days to the vesicles of *Herpes simplex* or *Herpes zoster*, but should be confined to skin, and not used for eyes.

Podophyllin (*Posalfilin*)
Used for anogenital warts (avoid in pregnancy, since it is teratogenic) and plantar warts. For plantar warts, a plaster with a central hole is first applied to protect surrounding skin. Formaldehyde or glutaraldehyde are also used.

Corticosteroids
These are used for eczematous conditions, when other treatments have failed. They suppress inflammation and symptoms, but these are likely to recur when treatment is stopped. Their use in minor or undiagnosed skin disorders is to be deprecated. Systemic side effects (Chapter 13) due to absorption can occur.

Local adverse effects. Exacerbation of skin infection, skin atrophy, hirsutism and acneiform rash, especially on the face.

Preparations
The weakest preparation which is effective should be used. Examples include: hydrocortisone (*Cortril, Efcortelan, Locoid*), beclomethasone (*Propaderm*), betamethasone (*Betnovate*), clobetasol (*Dermovate*), desonide (*Tridesilon*),

diflucortolone (*Temetex*), fluclorolone (*Topilar*), fluocinolone (*Synalar*), flucinonide (*Metosyn*), fluocortolone (*Ultradil*), flurandrenolone (*Haelan*), halcinonide (*Halciderm*) and triamcinolone (*Ledercort*).

There are many proprietary corticosteroid preparations combined with antibiotics. There is little, if any, indication for their use.

Preparations for specific skin conditions

Benzoyl peroxide (*Acnegel, Benoxyl*)
A skin-cleanser, used for acne.

Coal tar
Available also as zinc and coal tar, as a paste impregnated bandage, cream, lotion, shampoo and bath additive, for eczema and psoriasis. Can be unsightly.

Dithranol (*Dithrolan, Psoradrate*)
Lassar's paste (dithranol in zinc and salicylic acid), or dithranol alone, are used for psoriasis, applied daily, preferably after a coal-tar bath. Irritant to broken skin and eyes.

Ichthammol
A milder alternative to coal tar.

Resorcinol and sulphur paste
A peeling agent used for acne. Sulphur or zinc sulphide may also be used alone, but are less effective. Prolonged use of resorcinol can cause hypothyroidism.

Salicylic acid
A peeling agent, used for psoriasis and acne. *Aserbine* is a proprietary preparation, containing other acids in addition, used for desloughing wounds.

Urea (*Calmurid***)**
Has some effect in eczema.

Selenium sulphide (*Lenium, Selsun***)**
A shampoo, used for seborrheic dermatitis.

ANTISEPTICS AND DISINFECTANTS

Antiseptics are agents that inhibit the growth of micro-organisms. Disinfectants destroy organisms and their products which are capable of producing disease. A substance that may be used as a disinfectant in high concentration may have an antiseptic action in weaker concentration. Both are effective only for a limited time and above a certain concentration.

They are used for pre-operative skin sterilization, and for some infected skin conditions.

Coal tar derivatives
Phenol and cresol are disinfectants, too caustic to be used on skin.

Crystal Violet (Gentian Violet) and Brilliant Green are used for infected skin conditions.

Chloroxylenol solution (5%)
Used for skin cleaning. Less caustic than phenol, but may give rise to skin sensitivity. A similar proprietary preparation is *Dettol*.

Chlorhexidine (*Hibitane***)**
A widely used skin antiseptic. Inactivated by soap.

Hexachlorophane
Used in soap (*Sidal*) and in powder form (*Sterzac*), often for hand washing (*pHiso-Med*).

Oxidizing agents
These liberate oxygen on contact with organic matter and are used for cleaning infected wounds.

Hydrogen peroxide (*Hioxyl*)

Potassium permanganate
A dark purple crystalline solid which dissolves readily in water. It changes from pink/mauve to brown when oxygen is given off.

Silver nitrate
Can be used for infected wounds, but stains skin black. Toxic if used for more than a few days.

Reducing agents
Formaldehyde solution (*Formalin*)
It is a powerful antiseptic solution containing about 30% formaldehyde. It does not damage metals or fabrics and is used for sterilizing instruments.

Formalin is very irritant to the eyes and should not be used on tissues.

Solution of borax and formaldehyde (Instrument solution)
Used for storing surgical instruments. In a warm atmosphere, it liberates unpleasant fumes, and is liable to leave resinous deposits on the instruments.

Paraformaldehyde (*Paraform*)
A solidified form of formaldehyde. Used to fumigate sealed rooms.

The halogens
Chlorinated lime (bleaching powder)
Used as a disinfectant and may also be added to swimming-bath water.

Chlorinated lime and boric acid solution (*Eusol*)

Contains equal parts of each constituent. *Eusol* gives off chlorine which is antiseptic.

Used for irrigating wounds and cavities. It deteriorates after two weeks.

Sodium hydrochlorite solution (*Milton*)

An alkaline solution which is more stable than *Eusol*.

Indications are as for *Eusol*, and as a 1:80 solution for sterilizing infants' feeding bottles.

Iodine

Used as a skin antiseptic in a 1% or 2% alcohol or potassium iodide solution. Some people are sensitive to iodine and a skin test should be carried out before any large application.

Compound iodine paint (Mandl's paint)

Povidone–iodine (*Betadine*)

Povidone slowly liberates iodine when in contact with the skin and mucous membranes.

Used for pre-operative skin preparation, wound sterilization, and for *Herpes zoster* vesicles.

Cleaning agents

Substances included in this section may be described as '*surface acting* agents' and can lower surface tension, allowing grease to be dispersed. They are also bactericidal, and this dual action makes them suitable for cleaning infected areas. They are incompatible with soap.

Cetrimide (*Cetavlon*)

Savlon is a proprietary preparation of cetrimide 3% with chlorhexidine 0.3%. Used for pre-operative skin cleaning.

Benzalkonium chloride solution (*Roccal*)
Used to disinfect skin before surgery and obstetrics, a bladder irrigation and for soaking babies' sundries.

MISCELLANEOUS PREPARATIONS

Dextran beads. Absorb wound exudate (*Debrisan*).

Aluminium salts. Used to check excessive perspiration (*Anhydrol forte*).

Topical local anaesthetics (e.g. lignocaine**) and antihistamines**. Should be avoided, as they commonly cause skin hypersensitivity.

Camouflaging creams. Can be used to cover disfiguring skin lesions.

Sunscreens. Absorb ultraviolet light and are used to prevent photo-allergy and phototoxicity due to disease or drugs. Preparations include aminobenzoic acid, mexenone (*Uvistat*) and padimate (*Spectraban*).

23 Drugs Used in Tropical Medicine

THE TREATMENT OF MALARIA

Malaria is a protozoal disease caused by four species of *Plasmodium* and is transmitted to man by the female *Anopheles* mosquito. The sexual phase of its reproduction takes place in the mosquito, and the asexual phase in humans. Plasmodia injected into man are carried to the liver, where they multiply (the exo-erythrocytic stage). Later they enter the blood stream and erythrocytes, causing symptoms.

Particular antimalarial drugs affect either the erythrocytic or exo-erythrocytic stage, but not both.

Drugs such as chloroquine, acting on the erythrocytic stage, will control the disease, which may be sufficient in an endemic area. However, except for malignant tertian malaria due to *P. falcifarum*, eradication requires subsequent treatment with a drug acting on the exo-erythrocytic stage also, such as primaquine. Treatment of malignant tertian malaria (quinine may be more effective than chloroquine) is completed by a single dose of *Fansidar* (pyrimethamine + sufadoxine) or mefloquine.

Chemoprophylaxis is used for visitors to endemic areas, to prevent infection. It must be started before entering the area, and continued for four weeks after leaving. The choice of drugs depends on the resistance patterns of the Plasmodia in the area (contact the Bureau of Hygiene and Tropical Medicine in London).

Chloroquine (*Avloclor, Malarivon, Nivaquine*)
Prophylactic dose 400 mg orally weekly; therapeutic dose

600 mg, then 300 mg after six hours, then 300 mg daily for two days, orally. Parenteral preparations are available if necessary.

The drug of first choice for treatment, acting on the erythrocytic stage, and useful for prophylaxis. Also occasionally used for rheumatoid arthritis, systemic lupus and amoebiasis. Very slow renal elimination, but well-tolerated.

Adverse effects. Gastro-intestinal upsets, headache, pruritus, visual disturbances. Retinal damage can occur with prolonged high doses.

Hydroxychloroquine (*Plaquenil*) is similar.

Quinine
Initial dose 600 mg intravenously over four hours, 12-hourly, then 600 mg three times daily, orally, for severe falciparum malaria.

Indicated for the treatment of severe, or chloroquine-resistant, falciparum malaria. Also commonly used for the relief of night cramp (dose 300–600 mg at night).

Adverse effects. Dizziness, tinnitus, deafness, visual disturbances, thrombocytopaenia.

Mefloquine
Prophylactic dose 1 g orally monthly; therapeutic dose 1–1.5 g orally as a single oral dose.

A new drug, effective in falciparum malaria, as an alternative to, or, if severe, to follow, a short course of quinine.

Adverse effects. Gastro-intestinal upsets are common.

Proguanil (*Paludrine*)
Dose 100–200 mg daily as prophylaxis.

Well-tolerated, safe in pregnancy. Acts on erythrocytic stage. Some strains of malaria are resistant.

Amodiaquine
Dose 400 mg weekly as prophylaxis.
Similar to chloroquine.

Pyrimethamine (*Daraprim*)
Dose 25–50 mg weekly as prophylaxis.
May also be combined with sulfadoxine (*Fansidar*) or dapsone (*Maloprim*).
Slowly eliminated, effective against erythrocytic forms. *Fansidar* is also used as an alternative to, or following, quinine, in falciparum malaria, as a single dose (pyrimethamine 50 mg + sulfadoxine 1 g).

Adverse effects. May cause megaloblastic anaemia by interfering with folate metabolism (usually only apparent with pre-existing folate deficiency). Some patients lack the enzyme glucose-6-phosphate dehydrogenase (G6 PD) in their erythrocytes, which may haemolyse when given pyrimethamine.

Primaquine
Dose 15 mg daily for two weeks.
Effective against exo-erythrocytic forms of benign tertian malaria, and can be used to eradicate the parasites, following initial chloroquine treatment. Rapidly metabolized.

Adverse effects. May cause severe haemolysis in patients with G6 PD deficiency (which is common in Asian, African or Mediterranean races, who should be screened for this prior to treatment). May also occasionally cause other blood dyscrasias.

Trimethoprim (*Ipral, Monotrim, Syraprim, Trimopan***)**
An antibacterial agent (Chapter 16) which can be effective in
malaria prophylaxis.

THE TREATMENT OF LEISHMANIASIS

Leishmaniasis is a protozoal infection transmitted by sand-
flies. Different species cause cutaneous, mucocutaneous and
visceral (kala-azar) disease.

**Sodium stibogluconate (sodium antimony gluconate)
(***Pentostam***)**
Dose 200–600 mg daily intravenously or intramuscularly for
30 days.
   Discolouration of the solution indicates inactivation by
light.

Adverse effects. Gastro-intestinal upsets, arthralgia, rashes,
bradycardia, haemolytic anaemia.
   N-methylglucamine antimonate is a similar pentavalent
antimony compound. Other drugs occasionally used are
pentamidine, hydroxystilbamidine, urea stilbamine and the
antifungal drug amphotericin B.

THE TREATMENT OF TRYPANOSOMIASIS

Trypanosomes are protozoa, spread in Africa by the tsetse
fly, and involving the central nervous system, causing
sleeping sickness. American trypanosomiasis is spread by
certain bugs, and it also affects the heart (Chagas' disease).

Suramin
Dose up to 1 g intravenously weekly for six weeks, after a 200
mg test dose.

Only effective in early stages, prior to nervous system invasion. Excreted unchanged very slowly.

Adverse effects. Cardiovascular collapse may occur. Nephrotoxic—should be avoided in patients with renal disease.

Pentamidine
Dose 150–300 mg intramuscularly daily for up to ten days.
Only effective in early stages, and some strains are resistant.

Adverse effects. May cause hypotension or hypoglycaemia.

Melarsoprol (*Mel B*)
Given daily intravenously in three-day courses at weekly intervals, and a gradually increasing dosage.
Extremely irritant (use dry needles). Rapidly excreted. Effective after central nervous system involvement.

Adverse effects. Encephalopathy is especially common, which may be fatal.

Nifurtimox
Dose 10 mg/kg orally daily for four months.
The only effective drug for Chagas' disease, but only in the acute phase.

Adverse effects. Mainly gastro-intestinal, they are common and may be severe.

THE TREATMENT OF AMOEBIASIS

Amoebic dysentery is caused by the amoeba *Entamoeba histolytica*. Liver involvement results in abscesses.

Metronidazole (*Flagyl*)
Dose 800 mg three times daily for five days following a
course of diloxanide (*Furamide*).

Vomiting is common with the high doses needed in
amoebiasis. Tinidazole is similar to metronidazole. Metronidazole is also used for trichomoniasis, giardiasis and
anaerobic bacterial infections.

Diloxanide (*Furamide*)
Dose 500 mg three times daily orally for ten days.

Relatively non-toxic and most effective against amoebic
cysts. Therefore, used alone in chronic asymptomatic amoebic
dysentery, otherwise following metronidazole.

Emetine
Dose 60 mg intramuscularly for a few days (or Dihydroemetine
100 mg).

Adverse effects. Cardiotoxic and causes nausea. Now only
used in severe dysentery, together with metronidazole.

Other drugs
Tetracycline, chloroquine and di-iodohydroxyquinoline may
also be used in addition in severe dysentery.

THE TREATMENT OF SCHISTOSOMIASIS

Schistosomiasis (bilharzia) is acquired by contact with fresh
water containing the trematodes (flukes or flatworms) be-
longing to the genus *Schistosoma*. The infection is predominantly intestinal or urinary.

Niridazole (*Ambilhar*)
Dose 25 mg/kg orally daily in divided doses for one week.

It should be avoided in patients with hepatic schistosomiasis, who fail to metabolize the drug, resulting in psychosis, convulsions and vomiting.

Oxamniquin
Dose 25 mg/kg for three days.

Well-tolerated, even with hepatic involvement. The drug of choice for intestinal schistosomiasis (due to *S. mansoni*). Useful for mass treatment.

Metriphonate
Dose 10 mg/kg fortnightly for three doses.

Very well-tolerated, but only effective against urinary schistosomiasis (due to *S. haemotobium*), for which it is the preferred drug. Since it is cheap, it is useful for mass treatment.

Praziquantel
A single oral dose of 40 mg/kg is effective against all species. Well-tolerated, but may cause abdominal colic.

Hycanthone (*Etrenol*)
A single intramuscular dose of 3 mg/kg is effective, for *S. mansoni* or *S. haematobium*, but since it is hepatotoxic, it should be avoided if there is liver involvement.

Antimony sodium tartrate
Given parenterally by various regimens, usually to a total of 2 g.

Although this and other antimony preparations were the usual treatment for schistosomiasis, it has largely been superseded by the newer, less toxic preparations. It may still be used for *S. japonicum*, the most difficult schistosome to treat. Causes vomiting, diarrhoea and cardiotoxicity.

TREATMENT OF INTESTINAL WORM INFESTATION

The two main types of worm encountered are roundworm (nematodes) and tapeworm (cestodes).

Infection with tapeworms and some roundworms occurs by ingestion, whilst other roundworms penetrate the skin. Other tissues are invaded during the life cycle, extra-intestinal involvement being especially important with some worms (e.g. toxocariasis).

When there is infestation with multiple species, an anti-helminth should be chosen which is effective against all of them, if possible.

Piperazine salts (*Antepar, Ascalix, Pripsen*)
Dose equivalent to 4 g of hydrate as a single oral dose.

Occasionally produces ataxia and gastro-intestinal upset, but usually very well-tolerated. Effective against the common roundworm (*Ascaris*) and threadworms.

Levamisole
A single oral dose of 150 mg.

Very well-tolerated. Effective against *Ascaris*. Tetramisole is similar.

Pyrantel
A single oral dosage of 10 mg/kg, occasionally repeated in heavy infestations.

A very safe, broad-spectrum drug, effective against *Ascaris*, hookworms and threadworms.

Bephenium (*Alcapar*)
Dose equivalent to 2.5 g of the base as a single dose.

Less effective than other drugs against *Ascaris*, but particularly useful with associated hookworm infestation.

Adverse effects. Well-tolerated, but vomiting may occur if several doses are given, which may be required for the hookworm *Necator americanus.*

Mebendazole (*Vermox*)
Dose 100 mg twice-daily for three days.

Well-tolerated, and effective against most roundworms and tapeworms. Especially useful for mass therapy in endemic areas, with multiple infestations.

Thiabendazole (*Mintezol*)
Dose up to 50 mg/kg daily for three days. May need to be repeated.

It has a broad spectrum of activity against roundworms, including *Toxocara*, and is the most effective drug for *Strongyloides stercoralis.*

Adverse effects. May cause gastro-intestinal upsets and hypersensitivity reactions.

Tetrachloroethylene
This is best administered as a suspension to a fasting patient. Subsequently alcohol and fat should be avoided for three days, to reduce potential hepatotoxicity, but side effects are rare. Effective against hookworms, but avoid in the presence of untreated ascariasis, since it may cause their migration, resulting in intestinal obstruction. Otherwise it is well-tolerated.

Viprynium
A single dose of 5 mg/kg, repeated after one week if necessary.

Effective against threadworms, but stains the clothing.

Niclosamide (*Yomesan*)

Dose 2 g chewed and swallowed on an empty stomach. Several courses of treatment may be required.

The drug of choice for intestinal tapeworms, except possibly the pork tapeworm (*Taenia solium*), where release of ova may result in tissue invasion (cysticercosis). However, this risk can be minimized by purging with 30 ml. of magnesium sulphate two hours after treatment.

THE TREATMENT OF FILARIASIS

Filarial worms are transmitted by insect bites: *Wuchereria bancrofti* and *Brugia malayi* by mosquitoes, causing elephantiasis; *Loa loa* by horse flies causing subcutaneous swellings and *Onchocerca volvulus* by the black fly, causing blindness. Apart from the latter worm, which invades the connective tissue, the lympatics are primarily involved.

Diethylcarbamazine (*Banocide*)
The dose is gradually increased to 10 mg/kg in three divided doses for three weeks. The course may be repeated after a month.

This drug is effective against all filarial worms, but onchocerciasis may require four or more courses and may still relapse subsequently owing to resistance of the adult worms.

The drug causes headache and nausea, but hypersensitivity to the dead worms may occur, with exacerbation of the skin lesions, especially with onchocerciasis (Mazzotti reaction). Pretreatment with corticosteroids and antihistamines may reduce these reactions. Since chronic elephantiasis is due to fibrosis of the lymphatics, it will persist after the worms are killed.

Suramin
Effective against adult worms, but only given to serious cases

of onchocerciasis owing to its toxicity—repeated course of diethylcarbamazepine are often preferred. Dose as for trypanosomiasis, except that only 200 mg is given initially, and the dose increased by 200 mg at weekly intervals.

THE TREATMENT OF LEPROSY

Leprosy is caused by a bacterium, *Mycobacterium leprae*. The disease has two extreme forms: with little immunity and many bacilli (lepromatous or multibacillary), or with few bacilli owing to a marked immune reaction (tuberculoid or paucibacillary). Intermediate forms are common.

Paucibacillary disease is treated with dapsone 25–50 mg daily for 3–10 years.

The multibacillary disease is treated with three drugs initially, to prevent dapsone resistance: rifampicin 600 mg daily for four weeks, clofazimine 100 mg thrice-weekly for one year, and dapsone 50–100 mg daily for life.

Immunological reactions (lepra reactions) may occur in the paucibacillary disease, requiring corticosteroids. A different immunological reaction may occur in the multibacillary disease, requiring thalidomide (avoid in premenopausal women), high doses of clofazimine or corticosteroids.

Dapsone
Start therapy with lower doses, which may have to be used throughout if poorly tolerated. May cause haemolytic anaemia, sulphhaemoglobinaemia, agranulocytosis, a lepra reaction and, rarely, a cutaneous allergic reaction.

The drug is also used to treat dermatitis herpetiformis.

Clofazimine (*Lamprene*)
Well-tolerated but causes skin pigmentation.

Rifampicin (*Rifadin, Rimactane*)
More rapidly effective than dapsone or clofazimine, rendering

the multibacillary patient non-infective within two weeks. Also a drug of choice for tuberculosis. Its usefulness is limited by its high cost.

Adverse effects. Colours urine red, and causes hepatotoxicity.

24 Radiographic Contrast Media

Contrast media outline parts of the body which are normally lucent on X-ray, to help in X-ray diagnosis. With the availability of alternative non-invasive diagnostic methods, such as computerized X-ray tomography (CAT-scans), radioisotope scanning and ultrasound, there has been a decline in the use of some contrast media. However, contrast radiology is still the only satisfactory method to outline the gastro-intestinal tract. In other situations, contrast media contain iodine, all of which have the potential to produce allergies and anaphylaxis.

Gastro-intestinal tract

Barium sulphate
Barium sulphate can be given by mouth or rectum, and, since it is not absorbed, is non-toxic. The consistency required varies with the part to be examined. Often, an effervescent substance is given to produce a better outline of the mucosa (air-contrast study).

Gastrografin
An iodine-containing mixture of sodium and meglumine diatrizoate. It is preferable to barium, if a perforation of the gut is suspected, since it is absorbed from the peritoneum and excreted in the urine.

Gall-bladder

Ipodate
Dose 1.8 g.

An oral preparation; the sodium salt is given as capsules (*Biloptin*), the calcium salt as sachets (*Solu-Biloptin*), on the evening prior to X-ray. It is concentrated in the gall-bladder (oral cholecystogram).

Meglumine ioglycamide injection (*Biligram*)
Dose 30 ml. of a 35% aqueous solution.

Given by injection or infusion, and excreted in the bile, outlining the bile ducts (intravenous cholangiogram).

Respiratory tract

Propyliodine
Dose 12–18 ml. of an oily or aqueous solution.

Occasionally used to outline the bronchial tree.

Urinary and reproductive tract

Diatrizoate compounds (*Urografin*)
These are water-soluble solutions, containing iodine, in various proportions, as sodium and meglumine salts of diatrizoic acid. If given intravenously, they are rapidly excreted by the kidneys (intravenous urogram), but can also be given by a ureteric catheter (retrograde urogram). If injected through the uterine cervix, the female reproductive tract is outlined (hysterosalpingogram). The salivary ducts may be similarly outlined (sialogram).

Central nervous system

Metrizamide (*Amipaque*)
Dose 10 ml. intrathecally.

A non-ionic, but water-soluble, iodine-containing contrast medium, which is the least toxic for outlining the cerebral ventricles (ventriculography), and subarachnoid space (myelography). Also sometimes used with computerized tomography (CAT-scan). Metrizamide is eventually absorbed from the central nervous system. Headaches, nausea and fits occasionally occur. Oil-based iodine compounds such as iophendylate (*Myodil*) are not absorbed, are more toxic and now rarely used.

Cardiovascular system

Iothalamate compounds (*Conray*)
An ionic, water-soluble, iodine-containing contrast medium. The different preparations contain varying concentrations of the sodium and meglumine salts of iothalamate. Although they have properties similar to those of the diatrizoate compounds, they are usually preferred for arteriography and venography, where they are given as rapid bolus injections (often requiring a mechanical injector for arteriography).

Iodized oil fluid injection (*Lipiodol Ultra-Fluid*)
A combination of iodine with a poppy-seed oil extract. Hypersensitivity reactions are more common than with water-soluble contrast media, and intravascular injection could be dangerous owing to oil embolism. It has been used for sialography and hysterosalpingography, but is mainly used for lymphangiography. It is injected into a lymphatic, and may persist for several months in the lymph-nodes. Prior to injection, the lymphatics are identified by injecting a dye, such as Sulphan blue, subcutaneously—subsequent excretion of this will colour the urine blue.

25 The Treatment of Poisoning

Poisoning and drug overdosage, either accidental or intentional (usually self-administered), is now a common problem. Early institution of appropriate treatment may well be life-saving. The basic principles of treatment may be divided into four parts:

1. Supportive treatment, to keep the patient alive, is the most important.
2. Removal of the poison to prevent further absorption.
3. Hastening of elimination of the poison.
4. Use of a specific antidote.

SUPPORTIVE TREATMENT

The effects of most poisons and drugs are usually self-limiting, with complete recovery, provided that vital bodily functions are maintained, especially respiration.

Maintenance of ventilation
A clear airway must always be ensured in unconscious patients. In addition, artificial ventilation and oxygen may be necessary.

Drugs used in the treatment of poisoning
Drugs sometimes required in the symptomatic management of poisoned patients include:

244 Pharmacology for Nurses

Diazepam for delirium and convulsions
Diuretics for pulmonary oedema
Anti-arrhythmic drugs
Opiates for pain

Fluid and electrolyte replacement is rarely an urgent problem, but accurate fluid balance measurements should be made from the outset.

REMOVAL OF THE POISON

Poisons or corrosives on the skin should be washed off with cold water and contaminated clothing removed.

Poisons taken by mouth, unless trivial, should be removed by gastric lavage as soon as possible, to prevent further absorption, unless corrosives, petrol or paraffin have been taken. In young children, or if lavage is unavoidable or refused, emesis may be induced by ipecacuanha emetic mixture (paediatric), followed by a large tumbler of water, in the following doses:

Age 6–18 months: 10 ml.
Age 18 months–5 years: 15 ml.
Age 5–10 years: 30 ml.
Older than 10 years: 45–60 ml. depending on body weight.

This dosage can be repeated once after 20 min if necessary. Other emetics, such as saline, are dangerous and should not be used. Ipecacuanha must not be given to unconscious patients, or for corrosive poisoning, or paraffin or petrol poisoning.

Milk is often given to reduce mucosal irritation, caused by many household and industrial poisons.

INCREASE ELIMINATION OF POISON

Forced alkaline diuresis is commonly used for salicylate or

phenobarbitone poisoning, since the renal elimination of these drugs is increased by an alkaline urine. This is achieved by giving intravenous sodium bicarbonate (1.26%), together with dextrose, saline and potassium.

Other methods of active elimination, such as haemodialysis or haemoperfusion, are rarely indicated.

USE OF SPECIFIC ANTIDOTES

Most drugs do not have a specific antidote, and poisoning is managed with supportive measures only. Exceptions are:

Narcotics
Respiratory depression is reversed by naloxone (*Narcan*) (0.4–1.2 mg intravenously). Further doses may be needed.

Paracetamol (*Panadol*)
Severe, sometimes fatal, liver damage can occur following overdosage of 20 tablets (10 g) or more. Methionine (2.5 g orally) or acetylcysteine (*Parvolex*) (150 mg/kg intravenously over 15 min, followed by a slow infusion) are extremely effective antidotes, if given within eight hours of paracetamol ingestion.

The popular analgesic *Distalgesic* contains both a narcotic and paracetamol.

Cyanide
Cyanide poisoning is often not immediately fatal, and patients significantly poisoned should be given dicobalt edetate (*Kelocyanor*)—600 mg in 40 ml. intravenously followed by 50 ml. of 50% dextrose.

Iron salts
Serious poisoning is most commonly seen in children, who mistake their mothers' tablets for sweets. Iron is chelated by

desferrioxamine (*Desferal*) given intravenously and intramuscularly, which is excreted rapidly in the urine.

Other heavy metals
Dimercaprol (200 mg intramuscularly in repeated doses) is
used for poisoning by most heavy metals. Lead poisoning is
treated with disodium calcium edetate (*Ledclair*) or trisodium
edetate given by dilute intravenous infusion as necessary.
Penicillamine (*Cuprimine, Distamine*) (1 g orally daily) is
an alternative and is preferred for copper poisoning.

Organophosphorus insecticides
Prevent skin absorption. Excessive vagal activity (prevented
by atropine 2 mg intravenously half-hourly) and muscle
paralysis occur, since the hydrolysis of acetylcholine by
cholinesterase is inhibited. Pralidoxime reverses this inhibition,
if given within twelve hours.

Methanol
The oxidation to very toxic metabolites of both ethylene
glycol (in 'antifreeze') and methanol is slowed by ethanol
(enough to maintain the patient pleasantly intoxicated).

26 Intravenous Fluids and Nutrition

Plasma electrolytes refer to the salt constituents of plasma. Electrolyte solutions are given intravenously to meet normal body fluid requirements, when patients are unable to take these orally, such as post-operatively, or when rapid replacement is necessary, as in severe dehydration. Adequate sodium chloride and water can be absorbed orally, even in patients with diarrhoea, if given with dextrose. This has proved extremely valuable in children, especially where hospital facilities are not available.

Sodium chloride and dextrose oral powder (*Dioralyte*)
The powder is dissolved in the correct volume of freshly boiled and cooled water for oral administration.

INTRAVENOUS FLUIDS

Intravenous fluids should be administered slowly, except where there is a marked fluid or electrolyte deficit. Otherwise, fluid overload may precipitate pulmonary oedema, especially in the elderly and in patients with renal and cardiac failure.

Dextrose 5% intravenous infusion
Used to provide water without electrolytes. Although the dextrose (glucose) is subsequently metabolized, the solution has the same osmolality as normal plasma.

Stronger solutions of dextrose (10% or 20%) are available to provide dextrose as an energy source, but cause phlebitis if given into a peripheral vein.

Sodium chloride intravenous infusion (0.9%)
Often referred to as 'normal' saline, it is isotonic with plasma, and is used to replace sodium, chloride and water. Very occasionally, more or less concentrated solutions are indicated.

Potassium chloride solution (strong)
10%, 15% and 20% solutions are available. 1.5 g of potassium chloride is equivalent to 20 mmol each of K^+ and Cl^-. The normal daily intake is 80 mmol. Strong potassium chloride solutions are added to dextrose or sodium chloride infusions to correct or prevent hypokalaemia. Dangerous hyperkalaemia can occur in renal failure, or if potassium is administered too rapidly (no more than 20 mmol/hour).

Sodium chloride and dextrose intravenous infusion
The usual strength is 0.18% sodium chloride and 4% dextrose.
  Used to maintain sodium and water intake, e.g. post-operatively.

Potassium chloride, sodium chloride and dextrose intravenous infusion

Potassium chloride and dextrose intravenous infusion

Potassium chloride and sodium chloride intravenous infusion
These are the same concentrations of sodium chloride and dextrose as above, but containing 10–40 mmol potassium/l.

Sodium bicarbonate intravenous infusion
A strong solution (8.4%) is used to correct acidosis during cardiac arrest only, usually as 50 ml. boluses. A weaker solution (1.4%) is infused to correct metabolic acidosis in other situations or to induce an alkaline diuresis (e.g. in

salicylate poisoning). No drugs should be added to sodium
bicarbonate infusions.

Dextran intravenous infusion (*Lomodex, Rheomacrodex,
Macrodex, Dextraven***)**
Dextrans are polysaccharides; since they are slowly metabolized, they can be used to expand the vascular volume. They
also reduce viscosity and have been given in peripheral
vascular disease and venous thrombosis. They are numbered
according to the length of the molecule (40, 70, 110 or 150).
Dextran 40 is the smallest and may cause renal failure.

Gelatin (*Gelofusin, Haemaccel***)**
Similar properties and uses to dextrans.

Salt-poor albumin (*Buminate***)**
Can be used to treat hypoalbuminaemia, but it is expensive
and its effect is short-lived. Details of other plasma and blood
products can be obtained from the Blood Transfusion
Service.

Dialysis fluids
Special fluids are available for peritoneal dialysis.
    Electrolyte concentrates are available to dilute with water
for haemodialysis.

INTRAVENOUS ADDITIVES

Drugs are sometimes added to intravenous infusions, to
achieve a rapid effect or to maintain constant therapeutic
plasma concentrations. Drugs may be added to infusion
bottles, or given as a more concentrated solution by infusion
pump. Intermittent short-duration (e.g. 30 min) infusions can
be given by injection into a burette or via a small-volume

infusion fluid container connected by a Y-connection to the regular infusion.

Finally, bolus injections may be made into the rubber septum of the drip tubing (especially for irritant cytotoxic drugs).

Disadvantages

Bacterial contamination. This can be reduced by using a strict aseptic technique, or ready-prepared solutions (such as potassium chloride or lignocaine, in dextrose).

Instability. Many drugs are unstable or precipitate in intravenous fluids, especially if the infusion is prolonged. Dextrose or saline are the most suitable; drugs should never be added to bicarbonate solutions, blood, fat emulsions, amino-acid solutions or mannitol. After addition, solutions should be thoroughly mixed by shaking.

Drug interactions. Many drugs interact in solution so that either or both may be inactivated. Therefore, no more than one drug should be added to an infusion.

Rapid effect. Especially with intravenous boluses, too rapid administration may produce severe, immediate side effects (e.g. hypotension with anti-arrhythmic drugs).

Hypersensitivity reactions can be minimized by starting infusion of drugs likely to produce these reactions (such as iron-dextran) very slowly.

Intravenous additive policy

There should be local policies defining:

1. What special training is required for nurses allowed to add drugs to intravenous infusions.

2. Which drugs may be given intravenously by designated nurses.
3. Appropriate labelling of infusion fluids with additives.
4. Provision of information charts regarding compatible admixtures.

INTRAVENOUS FEEDING

Wherever possible, patients should be fed orally. If necessary, diets can be given by naso-gastric tubes. Occasionally, such as following extensive bowel resection or in prolonged ileus, intravenous feeding may be necessary by a central venous catheter. Except for certain nutritional additives, drugs should not be added, and the intravenous feeding line should be used for no other purpose.

Aims of intravenous nutrition

The aims are to maintain electrolytes and trace elements, to replace nitrogen losses with amino-acid solutions and to supply calories.

Calories are best provided as glucose solutions (e.g. *Glucoplex*). Although fat emulsions (e.g. *Intralipid*) also have a high calorie content, they are usually given only once weekly, to provide essential fatty acids. Amino-acid solutions (e.g. *Aminofusin, Aminoplex, Synthamin, Vamin*) are given with glucose for most efficient utilization. Hyperglycaemia, requiring insulin, may occur.

Appendix

This appendix includes the proprietary names of drugs in common use, together with their approved or other names and their pharmacological action or indication for use.

Proprietary Name	Approved Name	Pharmacological Action
Achromycin	Tetracycline	Antibiotic
Acnegel	Benzoyl peroxide	Treatment of acne
Acthar	Corticotrophin	Increases corticosteroid secretion
Actrapid MC	Neutral insulin	Hypoglycaemia
Adalat	Nifedipine	Treatment of angina
Adcortyl	Triamcinolone	Corticosteroid
Adriamycin	Doxorubicin	Cancer chemotherapy
Adsorbotear	Hypromellose	Artificial tears
Aerosporin	Polymyxin B sulphate	Antibiotic
Afrazine	Oxymetazoline	Nasal decongestant
Agarol	Phenolphthalein and Liquid paraffin	Aperient
Airbron	Acetylcysteine	Mucolytic
Albamycin	Novobiocin	Antibiotic
Albucid	Sulphacetamide	Sulphonamide
Alcobon	Flucytosine	Antifungal
Alcomicin	Gentamicin	Antibiotic
Alcopar	Bephenium	Antihelmintic
Aldactone A	Spironolactone	Diuretic
Aldomet	Methyldopa	Antihypertensive
Alkeran	Melphalan	Cancer chemotherapy
Alloferin	Alcuronium	Muscle relaxant
Aludrox	Aluminium hydroxide	Antacid

Proprietary Name	Approved Name	Pharmacological Action
Althesin	Alphaxolone and alphadolone	Intravenous anaesthetic
Ambilhar	Niridazole	Treatment of schistosomiasis
Amikin	Amikacin	Antibiotic
Aminofusin	Amino-acids	Intravenous feeding
Aminoplex	Amino-acids	Intravenous feeding
Amipaque	Metrizamide	X-ray contrast medium
Amoxil	Amoxycillin	Antibiotic
Anaflex	Polynoxylin	Antibiotic
Anafranil	Clomipramine	Antidepressant
Anapolon	Oxymetholone	Anabolic steroid
Androcur	Cyproterone	Androgen antagonist
Anhydrol Forte	Aluminium salts	Astringent
Anovlar-21		Oral contraceptive
Anquil	Benperidol	Tranquillizer
Antepar	Piperazine	Antihelmintic
Anthisan	Mepyramine	Antihistamine
Anturan	Sulphinpyrazone	Treatment of gout, antiplatelet drug
Apisate	Diethylpropion	Amphetamine
Apresoline	Hydrallazine	Vasodilator
Aprinox	Bendrofluazide	Diuretic
Aquamox	Quinethazone	Diuretic
Aramine	Metaraminol	Vasoconstrictor
Artane	Benzhexol	Treatment of parkinsonism
Ascabiol	Benzyl benzoate	Anti-parasitic
Ascalix	Piperazine	Antihelmintic
Aserbine	Salicylic Acid	Treatment of wounds and ulcers
Asilone	Dimethicone	Antacid
Aspirin	Acetylsalicyclic acid	Analgesic
AT 10	Dihydrotachysterol	Increases serum calcium
Atarax	Hydroxyzine	Tranquillizer
Atensine	Diazepam	Tranquillizer

Proprietary Name	Approved Name	Pharmacological Action
Ativan	Lorazepam	Tranquillizer
Atromid S	Clofibrate	Reduces hyperlipidaemia
Atrovent	Ipratropium	Anticholinergic bronchodilator
Aureomycin	Chlortetracycline	Antibiotic
Aventyl	Nortriptyline	Antidepressant
Avloclor	Chloroquine	Anti-malarial
Bactrim	Co-Trimoxazole	Antibiotic
Banocide	Diethylcarbamazine	Antihelmintic
Baycaron	Mefruside	Diuretic
Baypen	Mezlocillin	Antibiotic
Becotide	Beclomethasone	Corticosteroid
Benadryl	Diphenhydramine	Antihistamine
Benemid	Probenecid	Treatment of gout
Benoral	Benorylate	Analgesic
Benoxyl	Benzoyl peroxide	Treatment of acne
Benzedrine	Amphetamine	Stimulant
Benzoxinate	Oxbuprocaine	Ophthalmic anaesthetic
Benytrone	Oestradiol	Oestrogen
Berkmycen	Oxytetracycline	Antibiotic
Berkolol	Propranolol	Beta-blocker
Berkozide	Bendrofluazide	Diuretic
Berotec	Fenoterol	Bronchodilator
Beta-Cardone	Sotalol hydrochloride	Beta-blocker
Betadine	Povidone-Iodine	Antiseptic
Betaloc	Metoprolol	Cardioselective beta-blocker
Betim	Timolol maleate	Beta-blocker
Betnelan	Betamethasone	Corticosteroid
Betnesol	Betamethasone	Corticosteroid
Betnovate	Betamethasone	Corticosteroid
Bextasol	Betamethasone	Corticosteroid
Biligram	Meglumine ioglycamide	X-ray contrast medium
Biloptin	Sodium ipodate	X-ray contrast medium
Biogastrone	Carbenoxolone	Treatment of peptic ulcer
Bioral	Carbenoxolone	Treatment of aphthous ulcers

Proprietary Name	*Approved Name*	*Pharmacological Action*
Bisolvon	Bromhexine	Mucolytic
Blocadren	Timolol maleate	Beta-blocker
Bolvidon	Mianserin	Antidepressant
Bonjela	Choline salicylate	Treatment of aphthous ulcers
Bradilan	Nicofuranose	Peripheral vasodilator
Brevidil	Suxamethonium	Muscle relaxant
Brevinor		Oral contraceptive
Bricanyl	Terbutaline	Bronchodilator
Brietal	Methohexitone	Anaesthetic
Brinaldix	Clopamide	Diuretic
Bronchodil	Reproterol	Bronchodilator
Broxil	Phenethicillin	Antibiotic
Brufen	Ibuprofen	Anti-inflammatory analgesic
Buminate	Albumin	Albumin replacement
Burinex	Bumetanide	Diuretic
Buscopan	Hyoscine butylbromide	Anticholinergic
Butazolidin	Phenylbutazone	Anti-inflammatory analgesic
Cafergot	Ergotamine	Treatment of migraine
Calcitare	Calcitonin (porcine)	Treatment of Paget's disease
Calcium Leucovorin	Folinic Acid	Methotrexate antidote
Calmurid	Urea	Treatment of eczema
Calsynar	Calcitonin (salmon)	Treatment of Paget's disease
Calthor	Ciclacillin	Antibiotic
Camcolit	Lithium carbonate	Controls manic-depression
Canesten	Clotrimazole	Antifungal
Capastat	Capreomycin	Anti-tuberculous drug
Capoten	Captopril	Vasodilator
Cardiacap	Pentaerythritol tetranitrate	Treatment of angina

Proprietary Name	Approved Name	Pharmacological Action
Carylderm	Carbaryl	Antiparasitic
Catapres	Clonidine	Antihypertensive
Cedilanid	Lanatoside C	Cardiac glycoside
Cedocard	Isosorbide dinitrate	Treatment of angina
Celbenin	Methicillin	Antibiotic
Celevac	Methylcellulose	Laxative
Ceporex	Cephalexin	Antibiotic
Ceporin	Cephaloridine	Antibiotic
Cetavlon	Cetrimide	Antiseptic
Chendol	Chenodeoxycholic acid	Dissolves gallstones
Chenofalk	Chenodeoxycholic acid	Dissolves gallstones
Chloractil	Chlorpromazine	Tranquillizer
Chlorocain	Mepivacaine	Local anaesthetic
Chloromycetin	Chloramphenicol	Antibiotic
Chocovite	Calcium and vitamin D	Vitamin D replacement
Choledyl	Choline theophyllinate	Bronchodilator
Cicatrin	Neomycin	Topical antibacterial
Cidomycin	Gentamicin	Antibiotic
Citanest	Prilocaine	Local anaesthetic
Claforan	Cefotaxime	Antibiotic
Clinoril	Sulindac	Anti-inflammatory
Clopixol	Clopenthixol	Tranquillizer
Clomid	Clomiphene	Stimulates ovulation
Cobalin-H	Hydroxycobalamin	Vitamin B_{12} replacement
Codelcortone	Prednisolone	Corticosteroid
Cogentin	Benztropine	Anti-parkinsonian
Colestid	Colestipol	Hyperlipidaemia
Colifoam	Hydrocortisone foam	Inflammatory bowel disease
Colofac	Mebeverine	Antispasmodic
Colomycin	Colistin	Antibiotic
Concordin	Protriptyline	Antidepressant
Conova 30		Oral contraceptive
Conray	Iothalamate	X-ray contrast medium
Controvlar		Combined oestrogen/ progestogen

Proprietary Name	Approved Name	Pharmacological Action
Coptin	Co-Trimazine	Antibiotic
Cordaronex	Amiodarone	Anti-arrhythmic
Cordilox	Verapamil	Anti-arrhythmic
Corlan	Corticosteroid	Treatment of aphthous ulcers
Corsodyl	Chlorhexidine	Mouth wash
Cortelan	Cortisone	Glucocorticoid
Cortenema	Hydrocortisone enema	Inflammatory bowel disease
Cortistab	Cortisone	Glucocorticoid
Cortisyl	Cortisone	Glucocorticoid
Cortril	Hydrocortisone	Topical corticosteroid
Cosmegen Lyovac	Actinomycin D	Cancer chemotherapy
Cotazym	Pancreatin	Contains pancreatic enzymes
Crescormon	Growth hormone	Growth hormone replacement
Crystapen	Benzylpenicillin	Antibiotic
Cuprimine	Penicillamine	Excess copper removal
Cutisan	Triclocarban	Antibiotic
Cyclogest	Progesterone	Progestagen
Cycloprogynova		Combined oestrogen/ progestogen
Cyclospasmol	Cyclandelate	Peripheral vasodilator
Cyklokapron	Tranexamic acid	Antifibrinolytic
Cytosar	Cytarabine	Cancer chemotherapy
Daktarin	Miconazole	Antifungal
Dalacin C	Clindamycin	Antibiotic
Dalmane	Flurazepam	Anxiolytic
Danol	Danazol	Inhibits gonadotrophins
Daonil	Glibenclamide	Oral anti-diabetic
Daranide	Dichlorphenamide	Treatment of glaucoma
Daraprim	Pyrimethamine	Anti-malarial
Dartalan	Thiopropazate	Tranquillizer
DDAVP	Desmopressin	Anti-diuretic action
Debendox	Dicyclomine	Antispasmodic, antiemetic

Proprietary Name	*Approved Name*	*Pharmacological Action*
Debrisan	Dextran beads	Absorbs wound exudate
Decadron	Dexamethasone	Corticosteroid
Declinax	Debrisoquine	Anti-hypertensive
Decortisyl	Prednisone	Corticosteroid
Deltacortril	Prednisolone	Corticosteroid
Demulen-50		Oral contraceptive
Dendrid	Idoxuridine	Antiviral
De-Nol	Tripotassium dicitrato-bismuthate	Antacid
Depixol	Flupenthixol	Tranquillizer
Depo-Medrone	Methylprednisolone	Corticosteroid
Derbac	Malathion	Antiparasitic
Derbac Shampoo	Carbaryl	Antiparasitic
Dermonistat	Miconazole	Antifungal
Dermovate	Clobetasol	Topical corticosteroid
Deseril	Methysergide	Migraine prophylactic
Desferal	Desferrioxamine	Iron poisoning antidote
Destolit	Ursodeoxycholic acid	Dissolves gallstones
Dettol	Chloroxylenol	Skin disinfectant
Dexacortisyl	Dexamethasone	Corticosteroid
Dexedrine	Dexamphetamine	Amphetamine
Dextraven	Dextran	Reduces blood viscosity
DF 118	Dihydrocodeine	Analgesic
Diabinese	Chlorpropamide	Oral anti-diabetic
Diamicron	Gliclazide	Oral anti-diabetic
Diamox	Acetazolamide	Treatment of glaucoma
Dibenyline	Phenoxybenzamine	Peripheral vasodilator
Diconal	Dipipanone	Narcotic analgesic
Digitaline	Digitoxin	Cardiac glycoside
Dihydergot	Dihydroergotamine	Treatment of migraine
Dilantin	Phenytoin	Anticonvulsant
Dimelor	Acetoheximide	Oral anti-diabetic
Dindevan	Phenindione	Anticoagulant
Dioralyte	Sodium chloride and dextrose	Oral salt replacement
Direma	Hydrochlorothiazide	Diuretic

Proprietary Name	Approved Name	Pharmacological Action
Disipal	Orphenadrine	Treatment of parkinsonism
Disipidin	Posterior pituitary extract	Anti-diuretic action
Dispirin	Soluble aspirin	Analgesic
Distaclor	Cefaclor	Antibiotic
Distalgesic	Paracetamol and dextropropoxyphene	Analgesic
Distamine	Penicillamine	Excess copper removal
Dithrolan	Dithranol	Treatment of psoriasis
Diurexan	Xipamide	Diuretic
Dixarit	Clonidine	Treatment of migraine
Dolobid	Diflunisal	Anti-inflammatory analgesic
Dopram	Doxapram	Respiratory stimulant
Dorbanex	Danthron	Aperient
Doriden	Glutethimide	Hypnotic
Dozine	Chlorpromazine	Tranquillizer
Dramamine	Dimenhydrinate	Antihistamine
Droleptan	Droperidol	Tranquillizer
Dryptal	Frusemide	Diuretic
Dulcolax	Bisacodyl	Aperient
Duogastrone	Carbenoxolone	Treatment of duodenal ulcer
Duphalac	Lactulose	Aperient
Duphaston	Dydrogesterone	Progestogen
Durabolin	Nandrolone	Anabolic steroid
Duromine	Phentermine	Amphetamine
Duvadilan	Isoxsuprine	Peripheral vasodilator
Dyazide	Triamterene	Diuretic
Dytac	Triamterene	Diuretic
Dytide	Triamterene	Diuretic
Ecostatin	Econazole	Antifungal
Edecrin	Ethacrynic acid	Diuretic
Efcortelan	Hydrocortisone sodium succinate	Glucocorticoid

Proprietary Name	*Approved Name*	*Pharmacological Action*
Efcortesol	Hydrocortisone sodium phosphate	Glucocorticoid
Effergot	Ergotamine tartrate	Treatment of migraine
Eltroxin	Thyroxine	Thyroid replacement therapy
Eludril	Chlorhexidine	Mouth wash
Endoxana	Cyclophosphamide	Cancer chemotherapy
Enduron	Methyclothiazide	Diuretic
Enteromide	Calcium sulphaloxate	Sulphonamide
Entonox	Nitrous oxide, Oxygen	Inhalational analgesia
Epanutin	Phenytoin	Anti-convulsant
Epifrin	Adrenaline	Mydriatic
Epilim	Sodium valproate	Anti-convulsant
Epontol	Propanidid	Intravenous anaesthetic
Eppy	Adrenaline	Mydriatic
Epsikapron	Aminocaproic acid	Antifibrinolytic
Equanil	Meprobamate	Tranquillizer
Eradacin	Acrosoxacin	Antimicrobial
Eraldin	Practolol	Cardio-selective beta-blocker
Erycen	Erythromycin	Antibiotic
Erythrocin	Erythromycin	Antibiotic
Esbatal	Bethanidine	Antihypertensive
Eserine	Physostigmine	Miotic
Esidrex	Hydrochlorothiazide	Diuretic
Ethrane	Enflurane	Anaesthetic
Eudemine	Diazoxide	Hypotension; hyperglycaemia
Euglucon	Glibenclamide	Oral anti-diabetic
Eugynon		Oral contraceptive
Eurax	Crotamiton	Antiparasitic
Eusol	Chlorinated lime and Boric acid	Antiseptic
Evadyne	Butriptyline	Antidepressant
Extrenol	Hycanthone	Treatment of schistosomiasis

Proprietary Name	Approved Name	Pharmacological Action
Evipan	Hexobarbitone	Hypnotic
Fansidar	Pyrimethamine and Sulfadoxine	Anti-malarial
Fazadon	Fazadinium	Muscle relaxant
Fectrim	Co-Trimoxazole	Antibiotic
Feldene	Piroxicam	Anti-inflammatory analgesic
Femulen	Ethynodiol	Progestogen contraceptive
Fenopron	Fenoprofen	Anti-inflammatory analgesic
Fentazine	Perphenazine	Tranquillizer
Feospan	Ferrous sulphate	Iron replacement
Fergon	Ferrous gluconate	Iron replacement
Ferrogradumet	Ferrous sulphate	Iron replacement
Ferromyn	Ferrous succinate	Iron replacement
Fersamal	Ferrous fumarate	Iron replacement
Flagyl	Metronidazole	Amoebicide; anti-bacterial
Flamazine	Silver sulphadiazine	Antibiotic
Flaxedil	Gallamine	Muscle relaxant
Flenac	Fenclofenac	Anti-inflammatory analgesic
Florinef	Fludrocortisone	Mineralocorticoid
Floxapen	Flucloxacillin	Antibiotic
Fluothane	Halothane	Anaesthetic
Formalin	Formaldehyde	Reducing agent
Fortagesic	Pentazocine and Paracetamol	Analgesic
Fortral	Pentazocine	Narcotic analgesic
Framygen	Framycetin	Antibiotic
Frisium	Clobazam	Tranquillizer
Froben	Flurbiprofen	Anti-inflammatory analgesic
Frusetic	Frusemide	Diuretic
Frusid	Frusemide	Diuretic

Proprietary Name	*Approved Name*	*Pharmacological Action*
Fucidin	Sodium fusidate	Antibiotic
Fungilin	Amphotericin	Antifungal
Fungizone	Amphotericin	Antifungal
Furacin	Nitrofurazone	Antimicrobial
Furadantin	Nitrofurantoin	Antimicrobial
Furamide	Diloxanide	Amoebicide
Fybogel	Ispaghula	Aperient
Fybranta	Bran	Prevents constipation
Galfer	Ferrous fumarate	Iron replacement
Ganda	Guanethidine	Treatment of glaucoma
Gantrisin	Sulphafurazole	Sulphonamide
Gastrocote	Alginates	Antacid
Gaviscon	Alginates	Antacid
Gelofusin	Gelatin	Restores blood volume
Genticin	Gentamicin	Antibiotic
Gestanin	Allyloestrenol	Progestogen
Gestone	Progesterone	Progestogen
Gestone-Oral	Ethisterone	Progestogen
Glibenese	Glipizide	Oral anti-diabetic
Glucophage	Metformin	Oral anti-diabetic
Glucoplex	Glucose	Intravenous feeding
Glurenorm	Gliquidone	Oral anti-diabetic
Glutril	Glibornuride	Oral anti-diabetic
Gonadotraphon FSH	Menotrophin	Stimulates ovulation
Gonadotraphon LH	Chorionic gonadotrophin	Stimulates ovulation
Gondafon	Glimidine	Oral anti-diabetic
Graneodin	Neomycin	Antibiotic
Gyno-Pevaryl	Econazole Nitrate	Antifungal
Gynovlar 21		Oral contraceptive
Haelan	Flurandrenolone	Topical corticosteroid
Haemaccel	Gelatin	Restores blood volume
Halciderm	Halcinonide	Topical corticosteroid
Halcion	Triazolam	Hypnotic
Haldol	Haloperidol	Tranquilliser

Proprietary Name	*Approved Name*	*Pharmacological Action*
Harmogen	Piperazine oestrone	Oestrogen
Heminevrin	Chlormethiazole	Hypnotic; anti-convulsant
Herpid	Idoxuridine	Antiviral
Hexopal	Inositol nicotinate	Peripheral vasodilator
Hibitane	Chlorhexidine	Skin antiseptic
Hiprex	Hexamine	Antimicrobial
Hormonin	Oestriol	Oestrogen
HRF	Gonadotrophin releasing hormone	Test for hypopituitarism
Hydergine	Co-Dergocrine mesylate	Cerebral vasodilator
Hydrea	Hydroxyurea	Cancer chemotherapy
Hydrenox	Hydroflumethiazide	Diuretic
Hydrocortistab	Hydrocortisone	Glucocorticoid
Hydrocortone	Hydrocortisone	Glucocorticoid
Hydrosaluric	Hydrochlorothiazide	Diuretic
Hygroton	Chlorthalidone	Diuretic
Hypovase	Prazosin	Vasodilator
Hypurin Isophane	Isophane insulin	Hypoglycaemia
Hypurin Neutral	Neutral insulin	Hypoglycaemia
Hypurin Protamine Zinc	Protamine zinc insulin	Hypoglycaemia
Idoxene	Idoxuridine	Antiviral
Iduridin	Idoxuridine	Antiviral
Illosone	Erythromycin	Antibiotic
Imferon	Iron dextran	Iron replacement
Imodium	Loperamide	Anti-diarrhoeal
Imuran	Azathioprine	Immunosuppressant
Inderal	Propranolol	Beta-blocker
Indocid	Indomethacin	Anti-inflammatory analgesic
Initard 50/50	Insulin (50% neutral, 50% isophane)	Hypoglycaemia
Insulatard	Isophane insulin	Hypoglycaemia
Intal	Sodium cromoglycate	Asthma prophylaxis
Integrin	Oxypertine	Tranquilliser

Proprietary Name	Approved Name	Pharmacological Action
Intralipid	Fat emulsion	Intravenous feeding
Ipral	Trimethoprim	Antimicrobial
Ismelin	Guanethidine	Antihypertensive; treatment of glaucoma
Isogel	Ispaghula	Aperient
Isopto-Frin	Phenylephrine	Treatment of glaucoma
Isopto Plain	Hypromellose	Tear substitute
Isordil	Isosorbide dinitrate	Treatment of angina
Jectofer	Iron sorbitol	Iron deficiency
Jexin	Tubocurarine	Muscle relaxant
Kabinase	Streptokinase	Fibrinolytic
Kantrex	Kanamycin	Antibiotic
Kannasyn	Kanamycin	Antibiotic
Kefadol	Cephamandole	Antibiotic
Keflin	Cephalothin	Antibiotic
Kefzol	Cephazolin	Antibiotic
Kelfizine W	Sulphametopyrazine	Sulphonamide
Kelocyanor	Dicobalt edetate	Cyanide poisoning antidote
Kemadrine	Procyclidine	Anti-parkinsonian
Kenalog	Triamcinolone	Corticosteroid
Kerecid	Idoxuridine	Antiviral
Ketalar	Ketamine	Anaesthetic
Kinidine	Quinidine	Anti-arrhythmic
Konakion	Phytomenadione	Vitamin K; warfarin antagonist
Lamprene	Clofazimine	Treatment of leprosy
Lanoxin	Digoxin	Cardiac glycoside
Lanvis	Thioguanine	Cancer chemotherapy
Largactil	Chlorpromazine	Tranquillizer
Lasix	Frusemide	Diuretic
Ledclair	Disodium calcium edetate	Lead poisoning antidote
Ledercort	Triamcinolone	Corticosteroid
Lederfen	Fenbufen	Analgesic
Lederkyn	Sulphamethoxy-pyridazine	Sulphonamide

Proprietary Name	*Approved Name*	*Pharmacological Action*
Ledermycin	Demeclocycline	Antibiotic
Lederspan	Triamcinolone	Corticosteroid
Lenium	Selenium	Seborrhoeic dermatitis
Lentard MC	Lente insulin	Hypoglycaemia
Lentizol	Amitriptyline	Antidepressant
Leostrin 20		Oral contraceptive
Leukeran	Chlorambucil	Cancer chemotherapy
Librium	Chlordiazepoxide	Tranquillizer
Lidocaine	Lignocaine	Cardiac arrhythmias
Lidothesin	Lignocaine	Local anaesthetic
Lincocin	Lincomycin	Antibiotic
Lingraine	Ergotamine	Migraine
Lipiodol Ultra-fluid	Iodized poppy-seed oil	X-ray contrast medium
Liskonum	Lithium carbonate	Antidepressant
Locoid	Hydrocortisone	Topical corticosteroid
Logynon		Oral contraceptive
Lomodex	Dextran	Reduces blood viscosity
Lomotil	Diphenoxylate	Anti-diarrhoeal
Loniten	Minoxidil	Vasodilator
Lopresor	Metoprolol	Cardio-selective beta-blocker
Lorexane	Gamma benzene hexachloride	Antiparasitic
Macrodex	Dextran	Reduces blood viscosity
Madopar	Levodopa and Benserazide	Anti-parkinsonian
Madribon	Sulphadimethoxine	Sulphonamide
Malarivon	Chloroquine	Anti-malarial
Maloprim	Pyrimethamine and Dapsone	Anti-malarial
Mandelamine	Hexamine	Antimicrobial
Mandl's Paint	Compound Iodine Paint	Antiseptic
Marcain	Bupivacaine	Local anaesthetic
Marevan	Warfarin	Anticoagulant
Marplan	Isocarboxazid	Antidepressant

Proprietary Name	*Approved Name*	*Pharmacological Action*
Marsilid	Iproniazid	Antidepressant
Marzine	Cyclizine	Antihistamine, anti-emetic
Maxidex	Dexamethasone	Ophthalmic cortico-steroid
Maxolon	Metoclopramide	Antispasmodic and anti-emetic
Medomin	Heptabarbitone	Hypnotic
Medrone	Methylprednisolone	Corticosteroid
Mefoxin	Cefoxitin	Antibiotic
Megaclor	Clomocycline	Antibiotic
Melitase	Chlorpropamide	Oral anti-diabetic
Melleril	Thioridazine	Tranquillizer
Menophase		Combined oestrogen/progestogen
Mequitazine	Primalan	Antihistamine
Meralen	Flufenamic acid	Analgesic
Merbentyl	Dicyclomine	Anti-emetic
Merital	Nomifensine	Antidepressant
Mestinon	Pyridostigmine	Cholinesterase inhibitor
Metamucil	Ispaghula	Aperient
Metenix	Metolazone	Diuretic
Methrazone	Feprazone	Anti-inflammatory analgesic
Metopirone	Metyrapone	Inhibits cortisol synthesis
Metosyn	Flucinonide	Topical corticosteroid
Mexitil	Mexiletine	Anti-arrhythmic
Microgynon 30		Oral contraceptive
Micronor	Norethisterone	Progestogen contraceptive
Microval	Levonorgestrel	Progestogen contraceptive
Midamor	Amiloride	Diuretic
Migril	Ergotamine and Cyclizine	Treatment of migraine
Milton	Sodium hydrochlorite	Antiseptic

Proprietary Name	Approved Name	Pharmacological Action
Miltown	Meprobamate	Tranquillizer
Minidin	Quinidine	Anti-arrhythmic
Minilyn		Oral contraceptive
Minocin	Minocycline	Antibiotic
Minodiab	Glipizide	Oral anti-diabetic
Minovlar		Oral contraceptive
Mintezol	Thiabendazole	Anti-helmintic
Mithracin	Mithramycin	Cancer chemotherapy
Mixogen		Combined oestrogen/ progestogen
Mixtard 30/70	Insulin (30% neutral, 70% isophane)	Hypoglycaemia
Modecate	Fluphenazine	Tranquillizer
Moditen	Fluphenazine	Tranquillizer
Mogadon	Nitrazepam	Hypnotic
Molipaxin	Trazodone	Antidepressant
Monotard MC	Lente insulin	Hypoglycaemia
Multilind	Nystatin	Antifungal
Multivite	Vitamins A, B, C and D	Vitamin replacement
Myambutol	Ethambutol	Anti-tuberculous drug
Mycardol	Pentaerythritol tetra-nitrate	Treatment of angina
Mycivin	Lincomycin	Antibiotic
Myciguent	Neomycin	Antibiotic
Mycota	Zinc undecenoate	Antifungal
Mydriacyl	Tropicamide	Mydriatic
Mydrilate	Cyclopentolate	Mydriatic
Myleran	Busulphan	Cancer chemotherapy
Mynah	Ethambutol	Anti-tuberculous drug
Myocrisin	Sodium aurothiomalate	Rheumatoid arthritis
Myodil	Iophendylate	X-ray contrast medium
Myotonine	Bethanechol	Acetylcholine agonist
Mysoline	Primidone	Anticonvulsant
Mytelase	Ambenonium chloride	Cholinesterase inhibitor
Naprosyn	Naproxen	Anti-inflammatory analgesic

Proprietary Name	*Approved Name*	*Pharmacological Action*
Narcan	Naloxone	Opiate antagonist
Nardil	Phenelzine	Antidepressant
Natrilix	Indapamide	Diuretic
Natulan	Procarbazine	Cancer chemotherapy
Nebcin	Tobramycin	Antibiotic
Nefrolan	Clorexolone	Diuretic
Negram	Nalidixic acid	Antimicrobial
Nembutal	Pentobarbitone	Hypnotic
Neo-Cytamen	Hydroxycobalamin	Vitamin B_{12} replacement
Neogest	Norgestrel	Progestogen contraceptive
Neo-Mercazole	Carbimazole	Anti-thyroid
Neo-Naclex	Bendrofluazide	Diuretic
Neoplatin	Cisplatinum	Cancer chemotherapy
Neosporin	Neomycin	Antibiotic
Nephril	Polythiazide	Diuretic
Netillin	Netilmicin	Antibiotic
Neulactil	Pericyazine	Tranquillizer
Neulente	Lente insulin	Hypoglycaemia
Neuphane	Isophane insulin	Hypoglycaemia
Neusulin	Neutral insulin	Hypoglycaemia
Niferex	Polysaccharide-iron complex	Iron replacement
Nilevar	Norethandrolone	Anabolic steroid
Nipride	Sodium nitroprusside	Vasodilator
Nivemycin	Neomycin	Antibiotic
Nivaquine	Chloroquine	Anti-malarial
Nizoral	Ketoconazole	Antifungal
Nobrium	Medazepam	Tranquillizer
Nolvadex	Tamoxifen	Oestrogen antagonist
Noludar	Methyprylone	Hypnotic
Norgeston	Levonorgestrel	Progestogen contraceptive
Noriday	Norethisterone	Progestogen contraceptive
Norimin		Oral contraceptive

Proprietary Name	Approved Name	Pharmacological Action
Norinyl		Oral contraceptive
Norlestrin		Combined oestrogen/ progestogen
Normacol	Sterculia	Laxative
Normison	Temazepam	Hypnotic
Norpace	Disopyramide	Anti-arrhythmic
Norval	Mianserin	Antidepressant
Noxyflex	Noxythiolin	Antimicrobial
Numotac	Isoetharine	Bronchodilator
Nupercaine	Cinchocaine	Local anaesthetic
Nuso	Neutral insulin	Hypoglycaemia
Nutrizym	Pancreatin	Pancreatic enzymes
Nystan	Nystatin	Antifungal
Ocusol	Sulphacetamide	Antibiotic
Omnopon	Papaveretum	Narcotic analgesic
Oncovin	Vincristine	Cancer chemotherapy
One-alpha	Alpha-calcidol	Increases serum calcium
Operidine	Phenoperidine	Narcotic analgesic
Ophthaine	Proxymetacaine	Ophthalmic anaesthetic
Ophthalmadine	Idoxuridine	Anti-viral
Opilon	Thymoxamine	Peripheral vasodilator
Optimax	L-Tryptophan	Antidepressant
Orabase	Carboxymethylcellulose	Treatment of aphthous ulcers
Orabolin	Ethyloestrenol	Anabolic steroid
Oradexon	Dexamethasone	Corticosteroid
Orahesive	Carboxymethylcellulose	Treatment of aphthous ulcers
Orap	Pimozide	Tranquillizer
Oratrol	Dichlorphenamide	Treatment of glaucoma
Orbenin	Cloxacillin	Antibiotic
Orlest-21		Oral contraceptive
Orovite	Vitamins A, B, C and D	Vitamin replacement
Ortho-novin		Oral contraceptive

Proprietary Name	*Approved Name*	*Pharmacological Action*
Orudis	Ketoprofen	Anti-inflammatory analgesic
Otosporin	Neomycin, Polymyxin B and Hydrocortisone	Antibiotic ear drops
Otrivine	Xylometazoline	Nasal decongestant
Ovestin	Oestriol	Oestrogen
Ovol	Dicyclomine	Anti-emetic
Ovran		Oral contraceptive
Ovranette		Oral contraceptive
Ovulen 50		Oral contraceptive
Ovysmen		Oral contraceptive
Pacitron	L-Tryptophan	Antidepressant
Palaprin	Aloxiprin	Analgesic
Palfium	Dextromoramide	Narcotic analgesic
Paludrine	Proguanil	Anti-malarial
Panadol	Paracetamol	Analgesic
Pancrex	Pancreatin	Pancreatic enzymes
Paraform	Paraformaldehyde	Reducing agent
Parenterovite	Vitamins B and C	Vitamin replacement
Parlodel	Bromocriptine	Dopamine agonist
Parnate	Tranylcypromine	Antidepressant
Parvolex	Acetylcysteine	Paracetamol poisoning antidote
Pavulon	Pancuronium	Muscle relaxant
Penbritin	Ampicillin	Antibiotic
Penicillin V	Phenoxymethyl penicillin	Antibiotic
Penidural	Benzathine penicillin	Antibiotic
Penthrane	Methoxyflurane	Anaesthetic
Pentostam	Sodium stibogluconate	Treatment of leishmaniasis
Pentothal	Thiopentone	Intravenous anaesthetic
Pentovis	Quinestradol	Oestrogen
Percorten	Deoxycortone pivalate	Glucocorticoid
Pergonal	Menotrophin	Stimulates ovulation
Peritrate	Pentaerythritol tetranitrate	Treatment of angina

Proprietary Name	*Approved Name*	*Pharmacological Action*
Peroidin	Potassium perchlorate	Anti-thyroid
Persantin	Dipyridamole	Antiplatelet drug
Pertofran	Desipramine	Antidepressant
Pevaryl	Econazole	Antifungal
Pexid	Perhexiline	Treatment of angina
Phanodorm	Cyclobarbitone	Hypnotic
Phenergan	Promethazine	Antihistamine, anti-emetic
pHiso-Med	Hexachlorophane	Antiseptic
Phospholine Iodide	Ecothiopate	Miotic
Phyllocontin	Theophylline	Bronchodilator
Physeptone	Methadone	Narcotic analgesic
Pimafucin	Natamycin	Antifungal
Piriton	Chlorpheniramine	Antihistamine
Pitressin	Vasopressin	Anti-diuretic
Plaquenil	Hydroxychloroquine	Anti-malarial
Ponderax	Fenfluramine	Appetite suppressant
Pondocillin	Pivampicillin	Antibiotic
Ponoxylan	Polynoxylin	Antibiotic
Ponstan	Mefenamic acid	Analgesic
Polybactrin	Neomycin	Topical antibiotic
Posalfilin	Podophyllin	Antiviral
Pramidex	Tolbutamide	Oral anti-diabetic
Precortisyl	Prednisolone	Corticosteroid
Prednisol	Prednisolone	Corticosteroid
Predsol	Prednisolone	Corticosteroid
Prefrin	Phenylephrine	Treatment of glaucoma
Pregnyl	Chorionic gonadotrophin	Stimulates ovulation
Premarin	Conjugated equine oestrogens	Oestrogen
Prempak		Combined oestrogen/progestogen
Priadel	Lithium carbonate	Controls manic depression
Prioderm	Malathion	Anti-parasitic

Proprietary Name	*Approved Name*	*Pharmacological Action*
Primolut N	Norethisterone	Progestogen
Primoteston	Testosterone	Androgen
Pripsen	Piperazine	Anti-helmintic
Priscol	Tolazoline	Peripheral vasodilator
Pro-Banthine	Propantheline	Anticholinergic
Profasi	Chorionic gonadotrophin	Stimulates ovulation
Progestasert	Progesterone	Progestogen
Progynova	Oestradiol	Oestrogen
Proluton Depot	Hydroxyprogesterone	Progestogen
Prondol	Iprindole	Antidepressant
Pronestyl	Procainamide	Anti-arrhythmic
Propaderm	Beclomethasone	Topical corticosteroid
Prostigmin	Neostigmine	Cholinesterase inhibitor
Prostin E2	Dinoprostone	Induce labour or abortion
Prostin F2 Alpha	Dinoprost	Induce labour or abortion
Prothiaden	Dothiepin	Antidepressant
Provera	Medroxyprogesterone	Progestogen
Pro-viron	Mesterolone	Androgen
Psoradrate	Dithranol	Treatment of psoriasis
Pulmadil	Rimiterol	Bronchodilator
Puri-Nethol	Mercaptopurine	Cancer chemotherapy
Pyopen	Carbenicillin	Antibiotic
Pyrogastrone	Carbenoxolone	Ulcer healing
Quellada	Benzene Hexachloride	Anti-parasitic
Questran	Cholestyramine	Reduces hyperlipidaemia
Rapitard MC	Biphasic insulin	Hypoglycaemia
Rastinon	Tolbutamide	Oral anti-diabetic
Razoxin	Razoxane	Sensitizes tumours
Retcin	Erythromycin	Antibiotic
Redeptin	Fluspirilene	Tranquillizer
Relefact LH-RH	Gonadotrophin releasing agent	Test for hypopituitarism
Rheomacrodex	Dextran	Restoration of blood volume
Rheumox	Azapropazone	Anti-inflammatory analgesic

Proprietary Name	Approved Name	Pharmacological Action
Rhythmodan	Disopyramide	Anti-arrhythmic
Rifadin	Rifampicin	Anti-bacterial
Rimactane	Rifampicin	Anti-bacterial
Rivotril	Clonazepam	Anticonvulsant
Ro-A-Vit	Vitamin A	Vitamin A replacement
Rocaltrol	Calcitriol	Increases serum calcium
Roccal	Benzalkonium	Cleaning agent
Rogitine	Phentolamine	Alpha-blocker
Ronicol	Nicotinic acid	Peripheral vasodilator
Rondomycin	Methacycline	Antibiotic
Roter	Bismuth subnitrate	Antacid
Rynacrom	Sodium cromoglycate	Prevents rhinitis
Salazopyrin	Sulphasalazine	Treatment of ulcerative colitis
Saluric	Chlorothiazide	Diuretic
Sanomigran	Pizotifen	Treatment of migraine
Scoline	Suxamethonium	Muscle relaxant
Seconal	Quinalbarbitone	Hypnotic
Sectral	Acebutolol	Cardioselective beta-blocker
Securopen	Azlocillin	Antibiotic
Selexid	Pivmecillinam	Antibiotic
Selexidin	Mecillinam	Antibiotic
Selsun	Selenium	Treatment of seborrhoeic dermatitis
Semitard MC	Semilente insulin	Hypoglycaemia
Senokot	Senna	Laxative
Septrin	Co-Trimoxazole	Antibiotic
Serc	Betahistine	Antihistamine
Serenace	Haloperidol	Tranquillizer
Serpasil	Reserpine	Anti-hypertensive
Serenid-D	Oxazepam	Tranquillizer
Sidal	Hexachlorophane	Antiseptic
Simplene	Adrenaline	Treatment of glaucoma
Sinemet	Carbidopa and levodopa	Anti-parkinsonian
Sintisone	Prednisolone	Corticosteroid

Proprietary Name	*Approved Name*	*Pharmacological Action*
Sinequan	Doxepin	Antidepressant
Sodium Amytal	Amylobarbitone sodium	Hypnotic
Soframycin	Framycetin	Antibiotic
Sofra-Tulle	Framycetin	Antibiotic
Solu-Biloptin	Calcium ipodate	X-ray contrast medium
Solu-Cortef	Hydrocortisone sodium succinate	Glucocorticoid
Soneryl	Butobarbitone	Hypnotic
Sorbitrate	Isosorbide dinitrate	Treatment of angina
Sotacor	Sotalol	Beta-blocker
Sparine	Promazine	Tranquillizer
Spectraban	Padimate	Skin barrier
Stelazine	Trifluoperazine	Tranquillizer
Stemetil	Prochlorperazine	Anti-emetic
Sterzac	Hexachlorophane	Antiseptic
Streptase	Streptokinase	Fibrinolytic
Stromba	Stanozolol	Anabolic steroid
Stugeron	Cinnarizine	Antihistamine
Sulphamezathine	Sulphadimidine	Sulphonamide
Sulfamylon	Mafenide	Antibiotic
Surmontil	Trimipramine	Antidepressant
Sustanon	Testosterone	Androgen
Symmetrel	Amantadine	Anti-parkinsonian
Synacthen	Tetracosactrin	Increases corticosteroid secretion
Synalar	Fluocinolone	Topical corticosteroid
Synflex	Naproxen	Anti-inflammatory analgesic
Synthamin	Amino-acids	Intravenous feeding
Syntocinon	Oxytocin	Induces labour
Syntometrine	Ergometrine and Oxytocin	Uterine stimulant
Syntopressin	Lypressin	Anti-diuretic action
Syraprim	Trimethoprim	Anti-microbial
Sytron	Sodium iron edetate	Iron replacement
Tace	Chlorotrianisene	Oestrogen

Proprietary Name	Approved Name	Pharmacological Action
Tachyrol	Dihydrotachysterol	Increases serum calcium
Tagamet	Cimetidine	Histamine$_2$-antagonist
Talpen	Talampicillin	Antibiotic
Tanderil	Oxyphenbutazone	Anti-inflammatory analgesic
Taractan	Chlorprothixene	Tranquillizer
Tears Naturale	Hypromellose	Artificial tears
Teejel	Choline salicylate	Treatment of aphthous ulcers
Tegretol	Carbamazepine	Anti-convulsant
Temgesic	Buprenorphine	Narcotic analgesic
Temetex	Diflucortolone	Topical corticosteroid
Tenormin	Atenolol	Cardio-selective beta-blocker
Tensilon	Edrophonium	Cholinesterase inhibitor
Tenuate	Diethylpropion	Appetite suppressant
Terramycin	Tetracycline	Antibiotic
Tertroxin	Liothyronine	Thyroid replacement
Testoral Sublings	Testosterone	Androgen
Tetmosol	Monosulfiram	Antiparasitic
Tetralysal	Lymecycline	Antibiotic
Thalazole	Phthalylsulphathiazole	Sulphonamide
Thiazamide	Sulphathiazole	Sulphonamide
Ticar	Ticarcillin	Antibiotic
Timoptol	Timolol	Treatment of glaucoma
Tinaderm	Tolnaftate	Antifungal
Tineafax	Zinc undecenoate	Antifungal
Tofranil	Imipramine	Antidepressant
Tolanase	Tolazamide	Oral anti-diabetic
Topilar	Fluclorolone	Topical corticosteroid
Tranxene	Clorazepate	Tranquillizer
Trasicor	Oxprenolol	Beta-blocker
Trasylol	Aprotinin	Anti-fibrinolytic
Tridesilon	Desonide	Topical corticosteroid
Tridione	Troxidone	Anti-convulsant
Trilene·	Trichlorethylene	Anaesthetic

Proprietary Name	Approved Name	Pharmacological Action
Triludan	Terfenadine	Antihistamine
Trimopan	Trimethoprim	Anti-microbial
Trinitrine	Glyceryl trinitrate	Angina
Trinordiol		Oral contraceptive
Triplopen	Benethamine penicillin	Antibiotic
Trisequens		Combined oestrogen/progestogen
Trobicin	Spectinomycin	Antibiotic
Tubarine	Tubocurarine	Muscle relaxant
Tuinal	Quinalbarbitone and Amylobarbitone	Hypnotic
Tryptizol	Amitriptyline	Antidepressant
Ubretid	Distigmine	Cholinesterase inhibitor
Ultradil	Fluocortolone	Topical corticosteroid
Ultratard MC	Ultralente insulin	Hypoglycaemia
Ureaphil	Urea	Diuretic
Urelim	Ethebenecid	Gout
Urografin	Diatrizoate	X-ray contrast medium
Urolucosil	Sulphamethizole	Sulphonamide
Uticillin	Carfecillin	Antibiotic
Utovlan	Norethisterone	Progestogen
Uvistat	Mexenone	Sunscreen preparation
Vaginyl	Metronidazole	Anti-microbial
Valium	Diazepam	Anxiolytic, anti-convulsant and intravenous anaesthetic
Vamin	Amino-acids	Intravenous feeding
Valoid	Cyclizine	Anti-emetic
Vancocin	Vancomycin	Antibiotic
Variotin	Pecilocin	Antifungal
Vascardin	Isosorbide dinitrate	Treatment of angina
Vasculit	Bamethan sulphate	Vasodilator
Vasoxine	Methoxamine	Vasoconstrictor
Vatensol	Guanoclor	Anti-hypertensive
Velbe	Vinblastine	Cancer chemotherapy
Velosef	Cephazolin	Antibiotic

Proprietary Name	Approved Name	Pharmacological Action
Velosulin	Neutral insulin	Hypoglycaemia
Ventolin	Salbutamol	Bronchodilator
Vepesid	Etoposide	Cancer chemotherapy
Vermox	Mebendazole	Anti-helmintic
Vertigon	Prochlorperazine	Anti-emetic
Vibramycin	Doxycycline	Antibiotic
Vira-A	Vidarabine	Anti-viral
Virormone	Testosterone	Androgen
Virormone-Oral	Methyltestosterone	Androgen
Visken	Pindolol	Beta-blocker
Vivalan	Viloxazine	Antidepressant
Voltarol	Diclofenac	Anti-inflammatory analgesic
Welldorm	Dichloralphenazone	Hypnotic
Whitfield's Ointment	Benzoic acid compound	Anti-fungal
Xylocaine	Lignocaine	Anti-arrhythmic
Yomesan	Niclosamide	Anti-helmintic
Zaditen	Ketotifen	Asthma prophylaxis
Zantac	Ranitidine	$Histamine_2$-antagonist
Zarontin	Ethosuximide	Anticonvulsant
Zinacef	Cefuroxime	Antibiotic
Zinamide	Pyrazinamide	Anti-tuberculous
Zincfrin	Phenylephrine	Treatment of glaucoma
Zovirax	Acyclovir	Antiviral
Zyloric	Allopurinol	Reduces urate formation

Index